Practice-Oriented Nutrition Research

An Outcomes Measurement Approach

Carol S. Ireton-Jones, PhD, RD, LD, CNSD

Director, Nutrition Program Management
Coram Healthcare
Principal, Preferred Nutrition Therapists
Carrollton, Texas

Michele Morath Gottschlich, PhD, RD, LD, CNSD

Director, Nutrition Services
Cincinnati Burns Institute
Shriners Hospitals for Children
Adjunct Associate Professor
University of Cincinnati
Cincinnati, Ohio

Stacey J. Bell, DSc, RD

Instructor in Surgery
Harvard Medical School
Research Dietitian
Surgical Metabolism Laboratory
Beth Israel Deaconess Medical Center
Boston, Massachusetts

An Aspen Publication®

Aspen Publishers, Inc.
Gaithersburg, Maryland
1998

The authors have made every effort to ensure the accuracy of the information herein. However, appropriate information sources should be consulted, especially for new or unfamiliar procedures. It is the responsibility of every practitioner to evaluate the approriateness of a particular opinion in the context of actual clinical situations and with due considerations to new developments. Authors, editors, and the publisher cannot be held responsible for any typographical or others errors found in this book.

Aspen Publishers, Inc., is not affiliated with the American Society of Parenteral and Enteral Nutrition.

Library of Congress Cataloging-in-Publication Data

Ireton-Jones, Carol S.
Practice-oriented nutrition research: an outcomes measurement approach/Carol S. Ireton-Jones, Michele Morath Gottschlich, Stacey J. Bell.
p. cm.
Includes bibliographical references and index.
ISBN 0-8342-0885-7
1. Dietetics--Research--Methodology. 2. Nutrition--Research--Methodology. 3. Outcome assessment (Medical care) I. Gottschlich, Michele M. II. Bell, Stacey J. III. Title.
RM218.I74 1997
613.2'072--DC21 97-23618
CIP

Orders: (800) 638-8437
Customer Service: (800) 234-1660

About Aspen Publishers • For more than 35 years, Aspen has been a leading professional publisher in a variety of disciplines. Aspen's vast information resources are available in both print and electronic formats. We are committed to providing the highest quality information available in the most appropriate format for our customers. Visit Aspen's Internet site for more information resources, directories, articles, and a searchable version of Aspen's full catalog, including the most recent publications: **http://www.aspenpub.com**
Aspen Publishers, Inc. • The hallmark of quality in publishing
Member of the worldwide Wolters Kluwer group

Editorial Resources: Gregory M. Balas
Library of Congress Catalog Card Number: 97-23618
ISBN: 0-8342-0885-7

Printed in the United States of America

2 3 4 5

This book is dedicated to the clinicians who, in their daily practice, are searching to find the answers by asking the questions.

Table of Contents

Contributors

Jon T. Albrecht, RPh, BCNSP
Assistant Director of Pharmacy
  Services
Parkland Memorial Hospital
Dallas, Texas
Clinical Assistant Professor
College of Pharmacy
University of Texas
Austin, Texas

David Allen August, MD
Associate Professor of Surgery
Robert Wood Johnson Medical
  School/UMDNJ
Director, Nutrition Support Services
The Cancer Institute of New Jersey
New Brunswick, New Jersey

Stacey J. Bell, DSc, RD
Instructor in Surgery
Harvard Medical School
Research Dietitian
Surgical Metabolism Laboratory
Beth Israel Deaconess Medical
  Center
Boston, Massachusetts

Todd W. Canada, PharmD, BCNSP
Clinical Specialist II
Department of Pharmacy Services
Parkland Health & Hospital System
Dallas, Texas

Marsha Evans-Orr, RN, MS, CS
Zone Clinical Manager
Apria Healthcare, Inc.
Phoenix, Arizona

Judith A. Fish, MMSc, RD, CNSD
Nutrition Support Dietitian
Nutrition/Gastroenterology
Geisinger Medical Center
Danville, Pennsylvania

**Michele Morath Gottschlich, PhD,
  RD, LD, CNSD**
Director, Nutrition Services
Cincinnati Burns Institute
Shriners Hospitals for Children
Adjunct Associate Professor
University of Cincinnati
Cincinnati, Ohio

xi

Jeanette M. Hasse, PhD, RD, FADA, CNSD
Transplant Nutrition Specialist
Baylor Institute of Transplantation
  Sciences
Baylor University Medical Center
Dallas, Texas

Gordon L. Jensen, MD, PhD
Director, Section of Nutrition Support
Associate Physician
Department of Gastroenterology and
  Nutrition
Geisinger Medical Center
Danville, Pennsylvania

Carol S. Ireton-Jones, PhD, RD, LD, CNSD
Director, Nutrition Program
  Management
Coram Healthcare
Principal, Preferred Nutrition
  Therapists
Carrollton, Texas

James D. Jones, MS
Senior Member of Technical Staff
Texas Instruments, Inc.
Lewisville, Texas

Orlando C. Kirton, MD, FACS, FCCP, FCCM
Associate Professor of Surgery
University of Miami School
  of Medicine
Miami, Florida

Gordon S. Sacks, PharmD, BCNSP
Assistant Professor
University of Mississippi Medical
  Center
Department of Clinical Pharmacy
  Practice
Jackson, Mississippi

David V. Shatz, MD, FACS
Associate Professor of Surgery
University of Miami School of
  Medicine
Miami, Florida

Foreword

Although a number of books have been written which help guide researchers through the planning, design, and eventual completion of a research project, only a few of these books have focused on the unique research needs of the clinical nutrition researcher.

The present book was co-edited by 3 nutrition researchers who have worked successfully in the field of nutrition for a number of years. My involvement with the authors came primarily through interaction with Dr. Carol Ireton-Jones during her formative years as a graduate student. I was her research advisor during this time period and quickly learned that she approached nutrition research with keen insight and great passion. Carol never seemed to be afraid of research work like so many other graduate students are at the beginning of their studies. Perhaps most importantly, Carol was good at "making things happen." She could readily link members of the medical research community into a cohesive block and get things done. Although my level of interaction with the other two authors has been more limited, their national prominence in the field of nutrition leads me to believe that they possess similar leadership traits that allow them to understand the unique needs of nutrition research teams.

By bringing their talents together these authors have constructed a visionary book that is long overdue. With the current explosion of interest in the field of nutrition it is unfortunate that a number of highly capable members of clinical teams around the country have not chosen to enter the personally rewarding area of nutrition research. This book provides readers with step-by-step guidance that is necessary when one wants to establish a nutrition research project which is (a) well designed, (b) fundable, and (c) publishable. Case studies are also provided by highly successful researchers who give a "spin" to research which focuses on their own specialty areas (Medicine, Dietetics, Nursing and Pharmacy).

In closing I would like to state that this book is notable for its content and timelessness. Once it becomes an addition to one's personal library it will only increase in value over the years. Drs Ireton-Jones, Bell, and Gottschlich are to be commended for their efforts as co-editors, and the authors of each chapter are to be thanked for sharing their knowledge.

George U. Liepa, PhD, FACN
Professor and Department Head
Department of Human, Environmental & Consumer Resources
Eastern Michigan University
Ypsilanti, Michigan

Preface

My first small step into research came through a clinical situation where I was asked to provide nutrition data for a study that a physician colleague of mine was doing with data from two of my burn patients. I had been collecting clinical data to "make my point" regarding the patients' nutritional needs and this information added considerably to the completed study, and to this manuscript. After finishing all of the class work necessary to complete my master's degree in nutrition, it became time to really "do research," that is develop my thesis topic and collect data.

Nutrition is a huge field and I thought about what to study: cholesterol metabolism, attitudes toward dieting, obesity? The answer came from my own practice setting when I discovered the solution with Dr. Charles Baxter, the Director of the Parkland Hospital Burn Unit. I was having a problem with providing the enormous amounts of calories needed to burn patients. The patients not only were surviving, but also appeared to be thriving on fewer calories. Dr. Baxter challenged me to measure the patients' metabolic rates using indirect calorimetry. Suddenly, I had my research question (which needed to be refined) and my research methods (which I needed to learn how to do). My lifelong interest in research began.

Although I have worked in many different settings—academia, home care, private practice, and industry—research has always been a part of my practice and I believe it has enhanced my satisfaction with the profession. Certainly the satisfaction of figuring out why something happens that leads to improved nutrition care is gratifying.

Practice-Oriented Nutrition Research: An Outcomes Measurement Approach is the work of three nutrition researchers who did not actually start out as researchers but soon discovered that solving problems and asking questions is an integral part of health care and of delivering quality nutrition care. This book is designed to provide the framework and assistance needed by the practitioner to develop and complete research studies that will propel nutrition into the 21st century.

Carol S. Ireton-Jones, PhD, RD, LD, CNSD
Director, Nutrition Program Management
Coram Healthcare
Principal, Preferred Nutrition Therapists
Carrollton, Texas

Introduction

The greatest harm that can befall the profession of nutritional science is the loss of its research-based authority. We live in a time when powerful forces, driven largely by economic motives, ply public myths, fears, and false hopes. For these forces, nutritional misinformation is nothing more than a marketing tool, a way to promote a growing array of untested supplements, herbal remedies, and weight loss/control products and services.

More often than not, nutritional misinformation exaggerates potential benefits, minimizes risks, and presents false or misleading therapeutic claims. Always, it seeks to subvert the validity of rigorous scientific assessment, infiltrate popular culture, and replace the hypothesis testing of well-designed experiments with uncorroborated studies, anecdotal evidence, or testimonials.

Self-taught, poorly educated "nutritionists," influenced by misinformation, rationalize misinformation's use in counseling, and seek widespread public acceptance of faddish alternatives to scientifically tested products and ideas. Similarly, while public relations-based "grass roots" campaigns stir the ranks of the ill-informed, corporate lobbyists expand their influence at the federal, state, and local levels.

Lawmakers, for instance, waded through a deluge of fact and misinformation to shape the recently passed Dietary Supplement and Health Education Act (DSHEA). This legislation, though well-intended and potentially valuable, is exploited by unscrupulous supplement suppliers who suggest that the rigors of the scientific method do not apply to the safe and efficacious use of their products. As a result of their influence,

DSHEA even protects over-the-counter sales of Ecstasy and Herbal Phen-Fen—remedies that deliver a dose concentration of ephedra alkaloids found in ma haung.

As misinformation penetrates the highest levels of government, the distinctions between "barefoot nutritionists" and professionally trained, highly educated dietitians and researchers continue to blur. Meanwhile, the ongoing devaluation of science frees special interests to exert even greater control over resource allocation, regulatory guidelines, and other public policies.

We are entering an era in which nutrient science has the potential to play a major role in health promotion and disease prevention. Nevertheless, we remain hobbled by a gap between practice guidelines and scientific proof. The FDA has long required human clinical trials in drug development, and the science of medicine has already parlayed major industry and government support into significant evidence-based proof for many clinical practices. Since food development has only recently been held to similar FDA mandate, nutrition science has yet to collect the critical mass of research required to support its methods for preventing, diagnosing, and treating disease.

These opportunities alone make this book a timely and much-needed guide, a catalyst for the army of students, teachers, researchers, and practitioners who know that scientific methods are the only valid basis for the practices of nutritionists, food engineers, and bionutritionists. It is also a timely response to a commentary by Professor Johanna T. Dwyer, Dsc, RD, "Scientific underpinnings for the profession: dietitians in research," which ran in the June 1997 issue of the *Journal of the American Dietetic Association.*

In that article, Dwyer drew on qualifications for American Board of Nutrition candidates to describe the skills required to successfully plan and execute research projects, including knowledge evaluation, the use of evidence to formulate and test theories, rational coherence, and hypothesis testing. These processes, covered in detail within this book, give students, teachers, and researchers the tools they need to translate basic and applied biology into nutrition realities.

This book comes at a time of unusual opportunity; a time when the director of NIH as well as an NCI cancer prevention review group are defining the new ideas, concepts, and discoveries that will guide efforts to meet the challenges of health promotion and disease prevention/treatment in the 21st century.

Worthy approaches will be rigorous, multidisciplinary, and novel; focused on topics that address the most compelling areas of need, such as child health and infant mortality, genetic engineering of foods for an ever-growing world population, the development of functional foods, and the use of dietary supplements and food fortification. Researchers will use the latest technology to enhance communications, and establish long-distance, even international, collaborations.

Much remains to be learned about the role of nutrients in health and disease. For those who seek to expedite the transfer of good, new science into optimal public nutrition, this book charts the course. For all motivated students with a desire to experience the exciting world of nutrition research, it makes today's rich scientific environment all the more accessible.

George L. Blackburn, MD, PhD
Chief, Section of Surgical Nutrition
Department of Surgery
Beth Israel Deaconess Medical Center, West Campus
Boston, Massachusetts

PART I

How To Conduct Nutrition Research in Clinical Practice

CHAPTER 1

Getting Started in Research

Carol S. Ireton-Jones and Stacey J. Bell

INTRODUCTION

Research is defined as studious and critical inquiry and examination aimed at the discovery and interpretation of new knowledge or expansion on a topic or idea.[1] Unfortunately, clinicians often view research as an overwhelming or unattainable goal, even though most unknowingly perform research (perhaps using sound research methods) in their daily practice. Quality assurance, surveys, new product evaluation, and cost-containment projects are all examples of research. The purpose of these activities is to document "what works and what does not work," which answers particular research questions. Useful research studies may be done to substantiate other previous investigations. Cost-effectiveness studies and studies of various nutrition therapies are absolutely indispensable in substantiating the value of nutrition in the health care environment.

In an editorial on research in the *New England Journal of Medicine*, Dr. C. Ronald Kahn stated: "The first step in picking a research project is to understand what makes research 'good.'"[2] (p.330) A good research project should be well performed, use up-to-date technology, carefully analyze and accurately report the data, and appropriately deal with the ethical considerations associated with animals and humans when they are involved. An outstanding research project asks important questions, yields truly new knowledge, leads to new ways of thinking, and lays the foundation for other research in the field. Although these are major propositions for the new researcher, a good research project can be developed by keeping these points in mind when preparing and conducting any research endeavor, regardless of its size. Research in nutrition is a dynamic and ongoing process. The answers will never be completely known to the myriad of potential research questions that are asked by the various members of the nutritional health care team—dietitians, physicians, nurses, pharmacists, and others. The key to answering some of these questions is for clinicians to plan, organize, conduct, and communicate research project findings.

OUTCOMES RESEARCH

An outcome in the context of health care is the result of a health care process, system, or episode of care.[3,4] Outcomes research has been defined as the rigorous determination of what works in medical care and what does not.[5] The health care industry has been seeking outcomes data from nutrition care providers, and such data are necessary to show the value and worth of the nutrition care provided. (Chapter 6 covers this topic in more detail.) The purpose of outcomes research is to collect and analyze data to help patients, providers, payers, and administrators make informed choices regarding medical treatment and health care policy. In business terms, the value of the product provided by nutrition care professionals—that is, health care and, specifically, nutrition support—is equal to outcome. Outcomes research can objectively determine what benefits are received from sophisticated, costly, and potentially hazardous nutrition interventions. These outcome-related questions must deal with financial issues and clinical effectiveness. Outcomes studies must be done with great care. A quick and dirty look can be just as inappropriate as research with methodological problems (such as small subject numbers, selection bias, and inappropriate choice of outcomes measures).[5,6]

GETTING STARTED

There are several misconceptions about performing research and becoming a researcher. Many clinicians believe that a lab is necessary to do research including nutrition research. Although much significant nutrition research is conducted under laboratory conditions with animals and humans, most clinical research is conducted in the field. A clinician may not realize the vast potential for opportunity in the hospital, clinic, alternate-site, or home care setting. It is important to recognize that most health care professionals are already involved in research of some kind. For example, most health care professionals keep Kardex or patient care files to monitor trends or changes in patient care. This is "doing research." Another common misconception is that one must have a master's or doctoral degree to do research. This is not so. Most of the authors of this book began clinical research projects without advanced degrees. It is important to begin the inquiry realizing that new knowledge does not have to be a brand new discovery but can be an expansion on a topic or idea. Research does require a desire and dedication to find the answer to one's question.

The Right Stuff

It is important to be sure that the potential researcher has the "right stuff" for research. Stacey Bell defined three necessary characteristics of a researcher.[7]

- Be curious.
- Be self-critical.
- Know the literature.

First, one must be curious, asking why something occurs in clinical practice and what can be changed or how something can be made better. The clinician-researcher questions the prevailing standard and seeks to find the answer to the question. For example, do burn patients really require 5000 to 6000 kcal/day as they are calculated using the Curreri equation, when they survive and recover well when they receive only 4000 kcal/day?[8] This is a research question that was answered in a clinical setting that has made a significant impact in the care of burn patients.

Second, one must be self-critical and take criticism well. Although the research question proposed may be important to the clinician, there are several steps to be taken before beginning data collection. Each step requires careful critical evaluation and revision. This is particularly true in reading and rereading abstracts, paper drafts, and research proposals. The peer-review process can be helpful, but the researcher must be open to suggestions and objective, critical evaluation.

Third, the researcher must know the literature. Repeating a study for validation is good, but repeating a well-established study is boring and does not further knowledge. The novice researcher may be embarrassed—or worse—by failing to conduct a full review of the literature on the research topic.

Hypothesis Generation

There are many aspects of initiating and completing a research study. The novice researcher who has an idea often jumps into the research process without considering all of the facets of conducting a successful research study. All the elements of a research project should be considered in the development phase (see Exhibit 1–1).

The most important element of a research study is defining the research question or problem. The first part of the research process is formation of the idea, topic, or research question. Researchers can select a topic in a variety of ways including coming across evidence of a problem that needs to be solved, encountering unanswered questions in the literature, or personally experiencing situations leading to unanswered questions. Once a question or topic has been selected, it should be defined as precisely as

---

Exhibit 1–1 Elements of a Research Study

- the problem/topic or question
- specific aims of the study
- background and significance of the proposed study
- preliminary studies or pilot studies
- research design
  1. patient population, stratification, randomization
  2. justification of sample size
  3. study procedure
  4. methods
  5. human subject concerns (institutional review board)
- data analysis and interpretation
- budget
- time frame

possible. The question should not be too vague or too broad. It is helpful to determine what research has already been done on the topic to narrow or broaden the question (see Exhibit 1–2).

Exhibit 1–2 Examples of Research Questions

- *"What are the energy requirements of people with human immunodeficiency virus (HIV) infection?"* This question is too broad: "people" are not classified; just using HIV disease is not specific enough; and there is no information as to how energy requirements are determined.
- A review of literature will help refine this question to: *"What are the energy requirements of HIV-positive, asymptomatic males as determined by indirect calorimetry?"*

A complete review of literature on the research topic will make the researcher aware of studies that other researchers have done in the same topic area. Such a review may provide information about previous studies, theoretical issues related to the subject, and pertinent methodologies that may assist with a new study.

In summary, clinical research can and should be an integral part of clinical care. It is time-consuming but rewarding. Clinical research may be simple or complex. Kahn has defined the points for serious researchers to consider in picking a research project.[2] Researchers who are just getting started may find this list of pointers useful (see Exhibit 1–3).

THE PROTOCOL

Developing a Protocol

Protocol development follows hypothesis generation. Preparation of a written protocol is essential for two reasons. First, it gives the researchers a chance to think through all of the stages necessary to carry out the study. Talking about the study design with a colleague is not sufficient; it is necessary to write down the essential information in each section of the protocol to ensure that all aspects of the study are covered. The second

Exhibit 1–3 Ten Commandments for Picking a Research Project

I.	Anticipate the results before doing the study.
II.	Pick an area on the basis of interest of the outcomes.
III.	Look for an underoccupied niche that has potential.
IV.	Go to talks and read papers outside your area of interest.
V.	Build on a theme.
VI.	Find a balance between low-risk and high-risk projects but always include a high-risk, high-interest project in your portfolio.
VII.	Be prepared to pursue a project at any depth necessary.
VIII.	Differentiate yourself from your mentor.
IX.	Do not assume that outstanding or even good research is any easier than outstanding basic research.
X.	Focus, focus, focus.

Source: Data from C.R. Kahn, Sounding Board, *The New England Journal of Medicine*, Vol. 330, No. 21, pp. 1530–1533, © 1994, Massachusetts Medical Society.

reason for writing a protocol is to gain colleagues' support and criticism. This mentor or peer support is valuable in helping the researcher to focus and refine research efforts. Who are these mentors? Colleagues (members of the researcher's discipline or other disciplines), coworkers, former professors. Some researchers have been unable to identify a mentor in their area; therefore, four dietitian members of the American Society for Parenteral and Enteral Nutrition (ASPEN) developed the Dietitians' Research Support Group (DRSG) to help new researchers (predominantly dietitians) develop research questions, review protocols, and refine abstracts. The members of the ASPEN DRSG get numerous phone calls from potential researchers who want to discuss studies that they are considering doing. Of these telephone inquiries, 90% never materialize into anything. In contrast, those who use this support group in the correct way—that is, by submitting a written protocol—have nearly a 100% success rate in completing their studies.

The number of pages of a protocol varies. For the National Institutes of Health (NIH), the maximum number of pages is 25. It is highly unlikely that any funding agency would require a protocol that exceeds 25 pages. Most industry-funded protocols can adequately cover the necessary information in about 3 pages. Foundations and professional societies generally require between 3 and 25 pages. Although the suggested page length may vary, the essential components of the protocol do not vary. These components are discussed below.

Abstract

The abstract of the protocol should be written exactly how it will be written for a scientific meeting, minus the results and discussion section. Several sentences about the expected results and implications of these results should be included. For busy reviewers who want an "executive summary," the abstract plus the specific aims should be sufficient.

Specific Aims

The specific aims can be a substitute for the research question in protocol development. The specific aims section should never exceed one page. This section usually contains one or two short paragraphs about the background leading up to the development of the study. Next, the specific aims are listed numerically. Generally this list should not exceed three specific aims. In nutrition studies, for example, one or more of the specific aims may be related to dietary intake changes or to changes in body composition as a result of a particular intervention. One or two specific aims must be reserved for the actual intervention. Specific aims may be listed in complete sentences or phrases. Each aim is followed by a few sentences of elaboration. As an example, the specific aims from a research proposal by Dr. Jeanette Hasse, RD, are presented in Exhibit 1–4.

INTRODUCTION

The introduction consists of two parts: (1) *background*, which is a short review of the pertinent literature of what others have published on the subject; and (2) *supporting evidence*, which is a summary of relevant work published by the researcher or his or her coworkers. If the researcher has not yet published on this subject, other subjects about which the researcher has published may be woven into this section.

Exhibit 1–4 Sample Specific Aims from a Research Proposal

Title of proposal: Effect of Growth Hormone Therapy on Body Composition and Clinical Outcomes in Liver Transplant Recipients.

Specific aims: The hypothesis of this study is that providing growth hormone (GH) therapy with nutritional support to liver transplant recipients will improve lean body mass and clinical outcomes following transplantation. The effect of GH on body composition (nitrogen balance, body fat, bone density, total body water, extra- and intracellular water, midarm muscle circumference, triceps skinfold, hand grip strength) and clinical outcomes (infection, rejection, number of days on ventilator, intensive care unit length of stay, hospital length of stay) will be evaluated in 20 malnourished liver transplant recipients pretransplant and during the first three months of posttransplant.

Source: Copyright © Jeanette M. Hasse, PhD, RD, LD, FADA, CNSD.

For example, an experienced researcher submits a grant to NIH on the effects of fish oil in patients with colon cancer, but the researcher has studied colon cancer patients in a limited way. The researcher writes a couple of paragraphs in the supporting evidence section about his experience feeding fish oil to patients with acquired immune deficiency syndrome (AIDS). In this way, he demonstrates how he achieved good patient compliance by adding the fish oil into a food bar, and he describes how he verified that the fish oil was incorporated into the white blood cell membrane by measuring eicosanoid and cytokine release from these cells. Because these same techniques will be applied to the patients with colon cancer, this discussion is useful in this section of the proposal.

If the novice has not published at all, he or she should simply name this section "Introduction," without dividing it into two sections. Regardless of whether the researcher has published previously, there needs to be a current review of the literature. At the very least, it is necessary to search back 5 years in the literature on the subject. Using a computer program such as MEDLINE, this task is made easy (Chapter 9). However, the proposal should not include irrelevant articles; a few pithy ones are far better than an extensive discourse on the entire field of nutrition. If possible, include articles from peer-reviewed journals only. The "punch" gained from non–peer-reviewed articles is substantially less. For research proposals submitted to industry, this section need not be extensive. This is because the researcher has usually spoken to the research and development (R&D) department first, and an area of study should be clearly defined. It is desirable to include one or two review articles on the subject in the introduction. For the previously mentioned study protocol on colon cancer and fish oil, a few reviews on the potential benefits of fish oil in these populations should be included rather than reviews on the two subjects independently, which would result in an extremely lengthy section.

Engaging in discussion with a company may elicit a request for a proposal in which the researcher and the company have a mutual interest. For example, in a meeting with the head of R&D of a manufacturer, both the company and the researcher may express a similar interest in studying patients with pathogen-negative diarrhea. Thus, the introduction of the proposal would be very short and include information only about the number of patients to be followed, the patients' diagnoses, and the researcher's past experience in conducting clinical trials (ie, publication track record). This can be sufficient to assure the company that the researcher has successfully conducted studies in the past and that there will be sufficient numbers of patients for the research study or clinical trial.

Methods

The methods section has one major goal. If someone else follows exactly what is described in this section, they should get the identical results of the original researcher. If they do not, then the methods were not precise enough or there was a methodological error (ie, the procedures were not followed exactly).

When reading published articles, many readers may skip the methods section, jumping to the results to see what happened. However, it is very important to read the methods section first. This allows the reader to understand fully what was attempted and allows a better appreciation of the results. In addition, the methods section of other articles may provide the researcher with information on a more appropriate methodology for his or her own study.

It is important to be exact so that the research is useful and applicable. For example, a publication may be unclear whether a new liquid formulation is for patients with AIDS or for patients who are human immunodeficiency virus (HIV) positive (the criteria for AIDS and HIV infection are defined by the Centers for Disease Control and Prevention). The results section shows improvement in weight maintenance and a reduction in the number of hospitalizations for those who took the new diet; it is the reader's impression that the diet is being marketed to all patients with HIV infection, regardless of whether they meet the criteria for AIDS. However, from the methods section, it is clear that most of the patients included in the study were in the early stages of AIDS or at the end of the period that is considered to be the HIV-positive state. Therefore, the formulation should only be used for patients who fall into one of these two categories, not the entire spectrum of patients with HIV infection.

The methods section usually includes the following subheadings:

- patients and animals (see Chapter 9)
- diet or other interventions (eg, drug, procedure)
- procedures/measurements (eg, indirect calorimetry/blood, urine components)
- statistics (see Chapters 2 to 4).

Subjects: Human and Animals

For clinical studies, this section should list inclusion criteria and exclusion criteria. This seems to be the best system to achieve clarity as well as brevity. For example, Stacey Bell recently completed a clinical trial in patients with HIV infection that listed exclusion and inclusion criteria (see Exhibit 1–5).

Some of the criteria are obvious, but less obvious criteria are described below. First, the study measured the effect of dietary fish oil on cytokines in the body. There was evidence in the literature that homosexual males with HIV infection had significantly lower concentrations of cytokines than males who used intravenous drugs, regardless of whether the intravenous drug users were HIV seropositive. Thus, including patients who contract HIV infection from sexual transmission and intravenous drugs would undoubtedly affect the results. Homosexual males were studied because 90% of the patient population contracts HIV infection through sexual transmission. No women were included because there are no cytokine data available, and there were fewer women than men where the study was done. Second, patients could not use nonsteroidal anti-

Exhibit 1–5 Inclusion and Exclusion Criteria in a Clinical Trial of Dietary Fish Oil on Cytokines in Patients with HIV Infection

---

Inclusion Criteria

1. documented HIV seropositive
2. homosexual transmission of virus
3. male
4. CD4 counts between 200 and 500 cells/mm^3
5. willingness to take at least five food bars per day for six weeks and understanding of the informed consent

Exclusion Criteria

1. AIDS
2. history of or presently using intravenous drugs
3. active secondary infection or tumor
4. regular user of nonsteroidal anti-inflammatory drugs (NSAIDs)

Source: Reprinted with permission from S.J. Bell, S. Chavali, B.R. Bistrian, C. Connelly, T. Utsunomiya, R.A. Forse, Dietary fish oil and cytokine and eicosanoid production during human immundeficiency virus infection. *J Parent Ent Nutr*, 20:43–9, © 1996.

---

inflammatory drugs (NSAIDs) because these drugs reduce cytokine and eicosanoid production, just as fish oil does. Thus, if frequent users of these drugs were included, it would be impossible to know whether the fish oil or the NSAIDs were suppressing the production of these metabolites. Third, the presence of an active infection or tumor results in increased production of cytokines. By omitting these patients, the researchers were able to obtain as homogenous a group as possible. The more characteristics that the subjects have in common, the more likely that the full effect of the intervention can be captured. In addition, a homogenous study population increases the chances that, if the study were performed elsewhere, the results could be reproducible.

In addition to the inclusion/exclusion criteria, it is necessary to include a statement about where the clinician-researcher will seek patients who meet these criteria. It may be necessary to conduct a cursory investigation to see how many patients there are in the database of the site where patients will be recruited. This additional effort often helps to secure funding, because granting agencies prefer to fund studies that will be completed swiftly.

Animal studies usually include criteria about the breed, age, sex, and weight of the animals. Obviously, it is much easier to gain homogeneity using animals as subjects, but the question always remains—what will happen in the clinical setting. All clinical studies require that the patients or their designated guardian sign an informed consent. This requirement applies to patients who are randomized to one of two treatments. Moreover, any collection of data from a patient requires a consent, regardless of whether the patient is aware that data are being collected. In cases where patient care is not affected, an "expedited review" system is available from most institutional review boards (IRBs). Most IRB consent forms request inclusion and exclusion criteria. In fact, much of what is included in the methods section of a protocol is required by the IRB for reviewing the proposal. Issues related to human and animal IRB approval are discussed in Chapter 9.

Diets or Other Interventions

It is best to present the diet or other interventions in tabular form. This allows for easy comparison of treatments, and it encourages the researcher to think of the relevant components (eg, micronutrients) of the intervention, which may be overlooked if prose is used to describe the interventions. Certainly, the amount of diet and the frequency it is administered or taken must be described in detail. It is necessary to state the method of delivery of the diet: volitional (ie, oral diet) or nonvolitional (ie, tube-feeding diet).

Procedures/Measurements

This is a tedious section to write and an even more tedious section to read. The author of the protocol should take the view that it is impossible to provide too much detail. This section needs to be so precise that anyone could duplicate the study. For laboratory procedures, this includes a level of detail such as the temperature of the water bath; the name and location of the manufacturer of the various instruments used; revolution speed of the centrifuge; concentration of certain reagents; incubation time of the samples; and volume of blood obtained.

The same amount of tedium applies to clinical procedures. For example, the researcher should state exactly how calorie needs are calculated (based on actual or ideal weights), the name and manufacturer of the scale being used to weigh the patients, the type and model number of the feeding tube and pump used, and the type and test tube top color used for blood drawing. All of this information is needed in order to gain IRB approval and to conduct the study.

Statistics

The final section of the protocol should include some mention of the statistical tools used. This material is covered in Chapters 2 though 4.

Data Collection

Data collection procedures used by the investigator are very important, whether the data are collected by hand or by a sophisticated computer system. There are two rules of thumb in relation to data collection:

1. Develop a data collection sheet early in the research project.
2. Collect more data than appears required, because it is difficult to go back or recreate the research situation after the fact.

Chapter 9 discusses data management systems. Computerized data management systems allow easy transfer to statistical analysis programs, which decreases time and effort. Data collection can make or break a study. It must be accurate. To ensure accuracy, a second evaluation of the data at the time of data collection may be useful.

Funding of Research Protocols

Many high-quality studies can be accomplished without any additional funding. These mainly fall under the guise of a quality assurance project, which means that the work is done as part of the regular clinical duties. An example of a quality assurance project is an evaluation of patients' compliance with the physicians' diet orders (calories received/calories ordered × 100) following use of a new data collection form.[9] In this project, a new data collection form was placed in front of the patients' medical charts and the deviations from the caloric goals prominently displayed. Data on compliance were collected for 6 months prior to the introduction of the new form and 6 months after the forms were introduced. The compliance with caloric goals for the two periods was compared.

Other studies require financial support to cover such things as diets, blood tests, laboratory tests, and so forth. Remember, it is unethical to charge a blood test to a patient's insurance plan when the test is required for the study only. Sometimes, it may appear that a test is clinically relevant—say a CD4 count for an AIDS patient. However, if the test is only necessary for research purposes—such as at baseline, week 4, and week 8—then the cost of the test must not be charged to the patient's insurance.

Funding is available from a variety of sources. These include drug companies, governmental agencies, private foundations, and professional organizations. Although it may seem that receiving grant money is about as likely as winning the lottery, the same rules apply—if you don't play, you can't win. The chances of being funded are increased by having a good protocol, so the investment of time is worth it. Also, many protocols can be "recycled" until they are funded.

PRESENTATION AND PUBLICATION

The final component of research is communication of results. This may be done by submitting an abstract of the entire project including brief results for a local, national, or international meeting. Alternately, the results may be presented in written form. Good research should be published only in a peer-reviewed journal, which further provides substance to the research. The applicability of the results may be communicated in lay journals and publications, but the research itself should be published in a well-recognized publication. Chapter 7 covers this topic in detail.

Novice and experienced researchers are absolutely necessary to the field of nutrition as it continues to evolve. Only good research will survive. Researchers can begin by following the information provided in this chapter (see Exhibit 1–6).

Research is exciting, fun, frustrating, time consuming, and difficult. When it is done well, it is always rewarding.

Exhibit 1–6 Outline of a Research Proposal/Project

1. Find and refine the research question.
2. Develop the research protocol.
3. Develop the abstract of the research protocol.
4. Determine the specific aims.
5. Identify funding sources.
6. Include the following proposal components:
   - introduction
   - methods
     - patients and animals
     - procedures/measurements
   - data collection (Develop a data collection sheet or program.)
7. Analyze the data, using appropriate statistical analysis.
8. Communicate the results.

REFERENCES

1. *Merriam Webster's Collegiate Dictionary*, 10th ed. Springfield, MA: Merriam-Webster, Inc; 1996:995.
2. Kahn CR. Sounding board. Picking a research problem: The critical decision. *N Engl J Med.* 1994;330:1530–1553.
3. Merkens BJ. Measuring outcomes of nutrition intervention. *J Can Diet Assoc.* 1994;55:64–68.
4. Davies AR, Doyle MA, Lansky D, et al. Outcomes assessment in clinical settings: A consensus statement on principles and best practices in project management. *Joint Comm J Qual Improv.* 1994;20:6–16.
5. August DA. Outcomes research, nutrition support and nutrition care practice. *Top Clin Nutr.* 1995;10(4):1–16.
6. Owens DK, Nease RF. Development of outcome-based practice guidelines: A method for structuring problems and synthesizing evidence. *Joint Comm J Qual Improv.* 1993;19:248–263.
7. Bell SJ. Having the "right stuff" for doing research. *Nutr Clin Pract.* 1991;6:173–174.
8. Ireton CS, Turner WW, Hunt JL, Liepa GU. Evaluation of energy requirements in thermally injured patients. *J Am Diet Assoc.* 1986;86:331–333.
9. Bell SJ, Molnar JA, Krasker WS, Burke JF. Dietary compliance for pediatric burned patients. *J Am Diet Assoc.* 1984;84:1329–1333.

SUGGESTED READING

Chernoff R. Research agenda conference discussion papers: A summary. *J Am Diet Assoc.* 1993;93:1045–1049.

Gould R, Schanklin C, Canter D, Miller J. Stimulating research among dietetic students. *J Am Diet Assoc.* 1994;94:1103.

Monsen ER. Forces for research. *J Am Diet Assoc.* 1993;93:981–985.

Schmidt L. A new career path for dietitians: Study coordinators. *J Am Diet Assoc.* 1993;93:749–751.

CHAPTER 2

Overview of Statistics in Research

James D. Jones

"There are three kinds of lies: lies, damned lies and statistics."
Benjamin Disraeli (1804–1881), English statesman and author

Many people believe that statistics can be a misleading or manipulative tool that can support a predetermined conclusion. Although statistics may initially seem intimidating, this field plays a pivotal part in the logical interpretation of complex physical processes. Statistics can both describe the observed behavior of a subject and support broader conclusions based on the observations. The goal of this chapter is to impart a basic understanding of important statistical terms and methods used in research.

It is true that statistics used out of context can be misleading. For example, an advertisement that claims that four out of five doctors recommend a product can mislead a consumer because of the many factors that could have influenced the reported statistics (such as the particular doctors surveyed or the phrasing of the questions). Statistics are used in research to indicate what is quantitatively known about a particular subject and to help determine what conclusions can reasonably be drawn. The conclusions of a research effort must be based not only on the statistics but also on the underlying knowledge and judgment that reinforce the conclusion. Knowing the degree of certainty (or uncertainty) helps determine what conclusions may be drawn.

THE ROLE OF STATISTICS IN RESEARCH

Statistics are used extensively in medicine, government, business, insurance, engineering, manufacturing, marketing, and many other disciplines. The weather forecaster may state that there is a 40% chance of rain, based on climate conditions and weather models. The meteorologist is specifying the level of uncertainty in the forecast due to random factors and the limitations of the weather models. The latest unemployment figures are released periodically by the government. These figures are based on sampling a small segment of the population that files new claims, using statistics to project a national rate. Automobile insurance premiums are set by actuaries who compile statistics based on factors such as age, sex, location, and driving record. The actuaries consider the probability and cost of an accident occurring based on these variables. After (or during) an election, a winner is projected by pollsters who conduct exit interviews of a small fraction of the electorate. The projection is made by selecting a small, representative group of voters and forecasting a winner based on statistical principles. Experienced gamblers at Las Vegas are aware of statistical factors and the rules of probability and use them to minimize their losses (or occasionally to win) in the casinos. The casino operators have set the payouts and gaming rules based on established probability theory to favor the casino when large numbers of wagers are made. Researchers who calculate life expectancy base their figures on medical research data, the presence of risk factors such as smoking, and a knowledge of statistics.

The fields of probability and statistics complement one another. Probability is considered more theoretical and uses abstract concepts such as infinite population sizes. Statistics, on the other hand, is an application of probability to studies where measurements or observations are made on specific subjects. Statistical methods deal with data from finite populations and measurements of limited precision. Statistics are used in research as a tool to describe and thus help understand behaviors or tendencies of the subject being researched. Together, statistics and probability provide a quantitative way of analyzing random processes.

Research includes the measurement or observation of physical objects. These measurements could include, for example, the cholesterol level of a group of patients or the carbohydrate content of particular food products.

The set of objects being measured is referred to as the *population*. In the above cases, the populations are the patients and foods being studied; a population is not necessarily a group of people.

Statistics provide a way to both describe (descriptive statistics) and infer (inferential statistics) knowledge about a random process. *Descriptive statistics* summarize particular features measured over the entire population being studied. For example, descriptive statistics would be the average high-density lipoprotein and low-density lipoprotein cholesterol levels of all the patients in a study. Descriptive statistics pertain only to the population studied and do not make broader conclusions.

Inferential statistics allow the researcher to draw conclusions from a specific set of measurements using knowledge of probability. Inferential statistics are based on a subset of a population referred to as the population *sample*. A pharmaceutical company may claim that taking aspirin will reduce the risk of heart attack. The inferential statistics in this case are the probabilities of heart attack, with and without aspirin. The claim would be based on research of subjects studied over a period of time. The population sample in this case is the group of people who took part in the study. The sample can restrict the applicability of the study, so it must be as similar as possible to the entire population. Inferential statistics are used to make conclusions based on the likelihood that a particular outcome of a research study is the result of chance. Outcomes that are very unlikely to be the result of random variations are then associated with one or more possibly causal factors. This does not prove a cause-and-effect relationship, but when coupled with supporting scientific reasoning, it can make this claim more conclusive.

DESCRIPTIVE STATISTICS

Descriptive statistics generally characterize a variable in terms of typical values and variability. The following are commonly used descriptive statistics for samples of a random variable. These statistics are used for variables that have a specific numeric value such as serum albumin level or metabolic rate.

Measures of Central Tendency

The mean, median, and mode are called measures of central tendency, because they describe the tendency of a variable to center around a given value. Most studies include measurement of several variables, and it is desirable to have information on typical values measured.

Mean

The mean value is the average of all the measurements taken. The mean is useful in determining the value around which the data are grouped. The mean of a set of *n* measurements of a variable *x* is:

$$\overline{X} = \frac{1}{n} \sum_{i=1}^{N} x_i$$

where Σ indicates the sum of the values following it, and x_i indicates the individual measurements of *x*: x_1, x_2, x_3 . . . through x_n. The number of measurements, *n,* is the sample size.

Median

The median is the 50th percentile, the value above which half of the measurements lie and below which half of the measurements lie. The median is useful in cases where the mean is shifted due to one or more data points that are considered *outliers*. An outlier is a data point that is very much higher or lower than the others. The median is found by listing the data in ascending numerical order, counting halfway through the samples, and noting the value. (Note that if the number of samples *n* is an odd number, the median is the value of the "middle" sample; if *n* is an even number, the median is the average of the two values closest to the middle.) Statistics on family income in the United States is an example where the median is a better descriptor of the typical value than the mean. Because some families make significantly more money than most, the average (mean) income is above the point that is considered typical. Thus, the median family income is a more representative statistic than the mean family income.

Mode

The mode is the most commonly occurring value of the variable. The mode is usually more useful if there are only a small number of distinct values the measurements can take.

Measures of Variability

The variance, standard deviation, range, and percentiles are measures of variability, because they describe how widely the values vary.

Variance, Standard Deviation, and Standard Error

The variance is a measure of how widely the data are spread around the mean value; the standard deviation is the square root of the variance and is a more frequently used term because it is measured in the same units as the data. The standard error is a measure of how accurately a sample mean can estimate the true mean of a population.

The variance (s^2) of a set of n measurements of x is:

$$s^2 = \frac{1}{n} \sum_{i=1}^{N} (\overline{X} - x_i)^2$$

where $\overline{X}$ is the mean value.

The standard deviation (s) is the square root of the variance.

The standard error (SE) is defined as:

$$SE = \frac{s}{\sqrt{n}}$$

Calling it an error does not mean there is a mistake; the term is simply a standard measure of uncertainty in estimating the mean.

Range

The range is the interval spanning the minimum to maximum values. The range by itself is not a very useful statistic, but it bounds the extremes of the measurements.

Percentiles, Quartiles, and Quintiles

These measures indicate what percentage of the sample was measured below a given value. Quartiles indicate the values capturing 25%, 50%, and 75% of the samples. Quintiles indicate the points capturing 20%, 40%, 60%, and 80% of the samples.

Example: A group of female patients participating in a study are weighed. The weight values in kilograms (kg) for the patients (sorted in ascending order) are as follows:

49, 57, 61, 64, 67, 67, 67, 67, 71, 71, 85, 100, 105, 111, 137, 171

Some descriptive statistics for this sample are as follows:

Sample size = 16
Mean = 84.3 kg
Median = 67 kg
Mode = 67 kg
Standard deviation = 31.8 kg
Standard error = 7.9 kg
Range = 49–171 kg
Third quartile (or 75th percentile) = 100 kg

In describing the mean and standard deviation, it is customary to give the figures as mean ± standard deviation (in this case, 84.3 ± 31.8 kg).

Note that the sample contains outliers at the top end of the weight scale (at 137 and 171 kg). These cause the distribution to be *skewed,* or non-symmetrical. This example has a positive skew, because the mean is above the median. In this case, the median or mode values are more representative of the "typical" patient in the group. Note that the mode is not a good measure if the resolution of the data is small; if measured to tenths of a kg, the group of four points at 67 kg might instead be 66.8, 67.0, 67.1, and 67.3 kg. Measured at that resolution, there may not be any data points that exactly repeat.

Graphs

Frequently, a graph can reveal more about the character of the data than a simple statistical description. The most common graph is the histogram (also known as a frequency distribution), which plots the relative abundance of data occurring within certain intervals. A histogram is formed by dividing up the range of possible measurements into *bins* and counting how often a value falls into each of the bins. Using the above example of patient weight, the bins might be as follows. (Note the bins are mutually exclusive.)

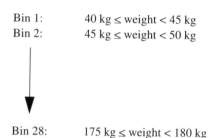

Bin 1:   40 kg ≤ weight < 45 kg
Bin 2:   45 kg ≤ weight < 50 kg

Bin 28:   175 kg ≤ weight < 180 kg

(Note the inequality signs, so that a given weight such as 45 kg that is near a bin boundary can fall into only one bin—in this case, bin 2.) For this example, the bins are 5-kg weight intervals, so *bin size* is 5 kg. To form a histogram, each patient weight is noted and a count is kept of how many patients fall into each bin. Selection of the bin size is important, and it may be necessary to determine this by trial and error. The bin size should be small enough to show the character and trends of the data, but not so small that there are excessive numbers of cells with zero counts. The graph shown in Figure 2–1 is based on the patient weights from the example and the bins described above. In this example, there were numerous bins with zero counts because the patient weights spanned a wide range with outliers.

The graph shows more clearly than the tabular data the character of the data, which is mostly clustered in the 55 to 75 kg range, but with several data points at much higher values. It also illustrates the skewed nature of the data; only 6 of the 16 data points are above the mean value. Also, the mode is clearly depicted; 4 of the data points fall into the 65 to 70 kg bin.

To underscore the utility of graphs, four histograms are presented in Figure 2–2. They all represent distributions with the same mean and standard deviation, but the shapes are clearly different. The likelihood of specific values occurring is quite different across these four distributions, a fact that cannot be conveyed by only the mean and standard deviation. Graphical summaries can often show more about the data than mean and standard deviation.

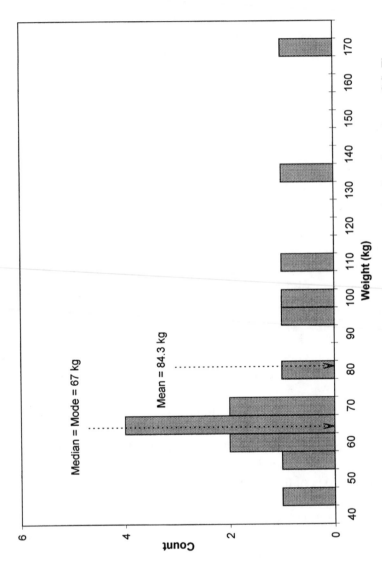

Figure 2–1 Histogram of female patient weights. *Source:* Reprinted with permission from Ireton-Jones, C.S. The energy equations: Development of equations for estimating energy expenditure in hospitalized patients, pp. 73–80, 1988, Graduate School of Texas Woman's University, Denton, Texas.

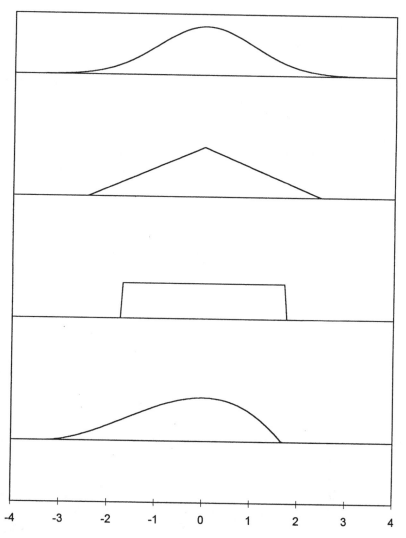

Figure 2–2 Different probability distributions with mean of 0 and standard deviation of 1.

Covariance and Correlation

There are also descriptive statistics to quantify the relationship of one variable to another variable. The most common such statistics are the *correlation* and *covariance*. Correlation (more commonly called the correlation coefficient) measures whether one variable increases, decreases, or is unaffected as the other variable increases. Covariance examines whether data from one variable are significantly separated from the mean at the same time that data from the other variable are significantly separated from the mean.

If different variables x and y are measured on the same n subjects and the individual measurements for the ith subject are x_i and y_i, the association between the two is called correlation. The correlation coefficient is

$$\rho = \frac{Cov\ (X, Y)}{s_X \times s_Y}$$

(where s_X and s_Y are the sample standard deviations for variables x and y, the covariance is

$$Cov\ (X, Y) = \frac{1}{N} \sum_{i=1}^{N} (x_i - \bar{X})(y_i - \bar{Y})$$

and $\bar{X}$ and $\bar{Y}$ are the sample means for the variables x and y.)

The correlation coefficient ranges from -1 to $+1$. A correlation near $+1$ indicates a strong positive correlation, meaning that increasing x values are associated closely with increasing values of y. A correlation near -1 also indicates a strong association, but decreasing y values occur as x increases. A correlation near 0 indicates that the values of x and y show little association.

Example: In a study of energy expenditure, the weight, age, and energy expenditure of patients are measured. The dietitian wishes to understand if the measured energy expenditure (MEE) is related to weight and age. In Table 2–1, data are recorded on 12 female patients (listed in order of increasing MEE to facilitate comparisons of MEE to age and weight). Larger MEEs tend to be associated with lower age or increasing weight. This data set has a correlation coefficient of 0.197 between energy expenditure and weight, indicating a slight positive correlation. The correlation

Table 2-1 Sample Data for Patient Measured Energy Expenditure, Age, and Weight

Patient No.	1	2	3	4	5	6	7	8	9	10	11	12
MEE (kcal/day)	1095	1157	1165	1200	1205	1422	1515	1549	1554	1599	1917	1980
Age	78	68	75	68	67	49	80	48	17	43	39	48
Weight (kg)	47	50	67	58	60	46	73	39	46	50	58	71

Source: Reprinted with permission from Ireton-Jones, C.S., The energy equations: Development of equations for estimating energy expenditure in hospitalized patients, pp. 73–80, 1988, Graduate School of Texas Woman's University, Denton, Texas.

coefficient between energy expenditure and age is –0.640, indicating a fairly strong negative correlation. Figure 2–3 illustrates the relationships between these variables. Figure 2–3A shows the relationship between energy expenditure and weight, with a small positive correlation as shown by the regression line. Figure 2–3B shows the relationship between energy expenditure and age, with a noticeable negative correlation.

INFERENTIAL STATISTICS AND HYPOTHESIS TESTING

The power of inferential statistics is their ability to suggest a conclusion that can be drawn about a population based on a sample of that population. Inferential statistical tests state and evaluate a *hypothesis*. A hypothesis is a theory or tentative explanation that accounts for a set of facts and can be tested by further investigation. The researcher phrases the research question in terms of a hypothesis supporting an expected conclusion. Measurements are then taken, and the hypothesis is tested and evaluated. Statistical tests by themselves do not prove a cause-and-effect relationship, but rather show whether observed results are unlikely to be the result of random variations.

As inferential statistics and hypothesis testing are discussed below, an example study is used to illustrate the concepts. The study involves a dietitian monitoring a diet and exercise program with the expectation of observing weight loss in the participants. It is a 6-week study of 14 subjects who show a weight loss of 6.55 ± 4.46 lbs (mean ± standard deviation) during the program.

Null and Alternative Hypotheses

Inferential statistics cannot always directly evaluate the research hypothesis but rather can test whether an opposite position (called the *null hypothesis*) is unlikely. The null hypothesis typically states that observed results are due to natural random variations that can exist in the sample being studied. The opposite position is the *alternative hypothesis*, which states that the results are not caused by random variations within the sample. A statistical analysis procedure states and tests the null hypothesis; if the null hypothesis is unlikely, it is rejected in favor of the alternative

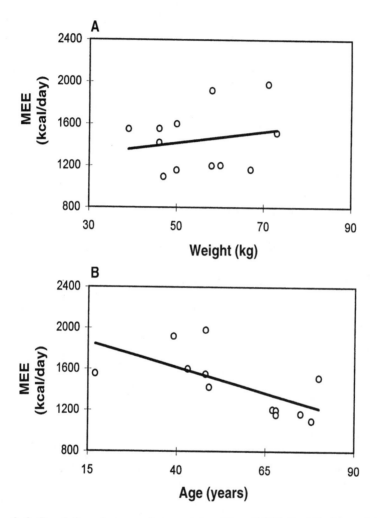

Figure 2–3 Correlation of measured energy expenditure (MEE) (kcal/day) to weight (kg) and age (years). (**A**) MEE versus weight, 12 subjects ($r = 0.197$). (**B**) MEE versus age, 12 subjects ($r = -0.640$). *Source:* Reprinted with permission from Ireton-Jones, C.S., The energy equations: Development of equations for estimating energy expenditure in hospitalized patients, pp. 73–80, 1988, Graduate School of Texas Woman's University, Denton, Texas.

hypothesis. (The null and alternative hypotheses are abbreviated as H_0 and H_a when stated as equations.)

For example, the dietitian conducting the diet and exercise program may state the hypothesis that the subjects will lose weight during the program; this becomes the alternative hypothesis. The null hypothesis is that the subjects will not actually lose weight during the program, meaning that any apparent weight loss is due to random variations (such as the variations in the scale used for weighing and normal physiological changes that cause a variation in weight). The statistical test would assess whether the null hypothesis—that the observed weight loss could be caused by random variations—is likely or unlikely. If the null hypothesis is unlikely, it is rejected and the researcher accepts the alternative hypothesis that the weight loss is *statistically significant*. This does not necessarily mean that the subjects lost a significant amount of weight (that is, enough to cause a change in their overall health status), but rather that the statistics conclusively demonstrated that weight loss occurred.

Significance Level and Power of Hypothesis Tests

In testing the null hypothesis, the *significance level* indicates how conclusive the result is. The significance level is the probability of incorrectly rejecting a null hypothesis that is actually true. The Greek symbol α is used to denote the significance level. Because the null hypothesis is considered an unlikely outcome, a significant result is declared when the probability is less than a small value (typically 5%). The notation $p < 0.05$ indicates that the probability, or *p-value*, of some event is less than 5%. In the diet and exercise program example, if the null hypothesis is rejected, this means that there is less than a 5% chance that the apparent weight loss is due to random variations. What constitutes a likely or unlikely result can depend on the nature of the research, so values of less than 5% may also be used. For example, if researchers are testing the safety of a drug or treatment regimen, a smaller significance level (0.01 or less) may be appropriate. Significance levels of above 5% are not usually considered conclusive.

Once the null and alternative hypotheses are defined, the desired significance level α is specified, and the appropriate type of statistical test is determined (Chapter 3 covers various statistical tests in detail). This results in *test statistics* being defined. The test statistics are the quantities that must be derived from the data to apply the chosen test method. In the diet and exercise program, the mean and standard deviation of subject weights before and after the study would be the test statistics. One of two equivalent options may then be chosen from this point to test the null hypothesis.

In the first option, a *critical value* (or values) is defined, which is the value of the test statistic at the given significance level. The experimentally determined value of the test statistic is compared to the critical value, and the null hypothesis is either rejected or accepted. If the null hypothesis is rejected, the result is considered significant and is annotated in the results (for an example where α is 0.05) as $p < 0.05$. In the example of the diet and exercise program, analysis of the subject weights indicates that a mean weight loss of at least 2.57 lbs is considered significant; this means that there is a 5% chance of observing a weight change of 2.57 lbs simply due to random variations when the subjects did not actually change weight. Because the actual mean weight loss was 6.55 lbs, the null hypothesis is rejected; the weight loss is statistically significant.

The second option explicitly calculates the *p*-value, the probability of the null hypothesis being true. If the *p*-value is less than α, the null hypothesis is rejected. In presenting results of the rejected null hypothesis for the second option (again, where α is 0.05), they may be stated as $p =$ (calculated value) or $p < 0.05$. In the diet and exercise program example, the *p*-value is calculated as $p = 0.00004$ and thus the weight loss is statistically significant.

Before the widespread use of computers, the first option was most common, because statistical tables contained critical values of the test statistic at common values of α (such as 0.01 and 0.05) and it was difficult to determine the actual *p*-value. Now the second option is often seen because the actual *p*-value can be calculated more easily, and knowing its exact value can be useful.

Hypothesis Testing

Hypothesis testing carries the risk of two main types of errors in drawing conclusions. A *type-I error* is rejection of a null hypothesis that is actually true. By definition, the probability of this error occurring is α, the chosen significance level (typically 5%). In the diet and exercise program example, there was a 0.004% chance of the apparent weight loss not being due to an actual weight loss; this *p*-value gives the researcher much more confidence in the conclusion than if it were closer to 5%. A *type-II error* is acceptance of a null hypothesis that is actually false, which occurs with a probability of β. The *power* of a test is equal to $1 - \beta$ and is the probability of correctly rejecting a false null hypothesis. In the diet and exercise program example, the probability of detecting a true loss in weight is $1 - \beta$. Determining the probability of a type-II error is not as simple as it is for a type-I error. The power of a statistical test to detect weight loss can be calculated for a specified amount of weight loss. The test will have a certain power for detecting a true weight loss of 6 lbs, for example, which will be greater than the power for detecting a weight loss of 4 lbs. The probabilities of both type-I and type-II errors can be managed by appropriate choice of sample size (see Chapter 4).

The combinations of hypothesis test results along with actual conditions and associated probabilities are summarized in Table 2–2.

OVERVIEW OF A STATISTICAL ANALYSIS PROCEDURE

This section outlines steps to define and conduct a research project that involves statistical data gathering and analysis. Parts of this process require a joint effort between researcher and statistician to ensure that the proper type and quantity of measurements or observations are made. The major steps in the process include the following:

1. Formulate the research question and hypotheses.
2. Design the experiment or survey.
3. Make observations or measurements.
4. Interpret the data.
5. Draw conclusions and document results.

Table 2–2 Decisions, Conditions, and Associated Probabilities in Hypothesis Testing

Decision	Actual Condition	
	Null Hypothesis True	*Null Hypothesis False*
Accept null hypothesis	Correct acceptance ($p = 1 - \alpha$)	Type-II error ($p = \beta$)
Reject null hypothesis	Type-I error ($p = \alpha$)	Correct rejection ($p = 1 - \beta$)

Most of this process is based on common sense and methodical scientific processes.

Formulate the Research Question and Hypotheses

Formulating a concise statement of the research objectives is essential and must capture the key principles behind the study. This form of problem statement is similar to what is required for writing a research abstract. A specific and quantitative definition of the research question will form the basis of the null and alternative hypotheses. Although the hypotheses can be refined and updated as the research proposal or pilot study progresses, a clear direction at the outset is necessary.

Design the Experiment or Survey

The next step is precisely defining the nature of the experiment or survey to test the research hypothesis. An *experiment* examines a population sample that is treated or controlled in some manner by the researcher. A *survey* examines a characteristic of subjects without altering or influencing those being studied. This step defines the variables of interest to be measured, and the method and frequency of measurement. The definition must be detailed enough that another researcher could replicate the study for a comparison of results. This step also identifies the portion of the population of interest to be included in the study. The population sample selected can be:

- *Random:* For statistical inference techniques to apply, the sample must be randomly selected. Methods of random sampling are discussed in Chapter 4.
- *Representative:* For any inferences to be valid, the population sample must adequately represent some larger population to which the inference will be extended.
- *Sufficiently large:* Sample size is critical to balance considerations of statistical confidence, probability of statistical error, and the size of the effort. Guidelines for sample size are discussed in Chapter 4.

- *Controlled for extraneous variables:* Understanding and eliminating (or accounting for) factors that could influence the measurements are critical to avoid false conclusions that omit a key variable.

The test statistics and methods to test the hypothesis must also be stated so that the appropriate data are gathered. The test statistics are needed to support the hypothesis testing, using the prescribed method (such as *t*-tests, analysis of variance, or correlation analysis). The desired significance level and power of the hypothesis testing should also be defined at this stage.

Additional steps that may occur here include defining criteria for subjects or data points to be included in the study and the length of the study. Defining the conditions for data validity at this stage simplifies questions that may arise later regarding the exclusion of apparently abnormal or nonapplicable data points. The duration of the study should also be defined, because the researcher should understand whether the subjects were examined or treated for a long enough period to yield statistically significant results. For example, a study on the effect of diet and exercise on cholesterol levels should have some minimum length required for the regimen to have a noticeable effect on the patients.

Make Observations or Measurements

Once the data requirements are defined, the measurements are compiled according to the research protocol. The researcher must maintain a rigorous record of the measurements and must perform and record appropriate equipment calibration to avoid introducing bias into the data. As measurements are made, they may be examined for outliers or abnormalities that would cause them to be excluded from the study. However, the researcher must keep all measurements, even if they are excluded from analysis. During a pilot study, initial data analysis may begin at this point if questions arise on the direction the research should take or if more or different data must be collected.

Interpret the Data

Data interpretation may begin during or after the data gathering phase. Tabulations or graphical summaries of the data assist in understanding the behavior of the subjects. It may be necessary to evaluate the data before hypothesis testing to ensure that data conform to the assumptions required by that technique (such as identifying outliers, defining normality or equality of variances). The values of the test statistics are calculated and the *p*-values compared to the defined significance level to test the research hypothesis. The data may warrant closer review in order to investigate the strength of cause-and-effect relationships that may explain the results.

Draw Conclusions and Document Results

The final step requires an integration of the statistical analysis with the underlying rationale that supports the findings of the study. Statistical results alone are not meaningful unless supported by deductive reasoning that explains the tendencies or behavior of the research subjects. If the *p*-value is close to the significance level, it may be necessary to address the possibility of a type-I error (if the null hypothesis is rejected) or type-II error (if the null hypothesis is accepted). Final documentation of results should be concise and quantitative, and graphical or tabular summaries should be used to illustrate key points of the study. The conclusions should clarify whether the findings are applicable to certain populations and conditions or exclude particular populations or conditions. If certain patients or subjects were excluded from the study, the researcher should justify this action and, if necessary, describe any effect this had on the statistical results. The researcher should consider some level of critical peer review before publishing or presenting results. Such a review takes time but can prove valuable by highlighting potential oversights, reinforcing the conclusions, or improving the clarity of the documentation.

Research articles published in scientific journals typically present a summary of the analysis after the abstract and introduction in a "Subjects and Methods" or similarly titled section. This section describes the experimental design, population groups studied, and research protocol, and it summarizes the statistical approach. The statistical approach may be introduced in a "Statistical Analysis," "Data Analysis," or similarly titled subsection. This subsection describes the statistical techniques used, key variables measured, and the specified significance level; it may state which analysis software package was used. Further presentation of the data and statistical findings occurs throughout subsequent "Results" and "Discussion" sections.

SUMMARY

A wealth of statistical techniques exists to support the analysis and expression of research findings. Descriptive statistics usually convey information about typical values and variability of the data collected. Inferential statistics assist in determining the significance of findings and extending conclusions to a broader population group. When conducting a research project that involves statistical data gathering and analysis, the researcher must follow these steps: (1) formulate the research questions and hypotheses; (2) design the experiment or survey; (3) make observations or measurements; (4) interpret the data; (5) draw conclusions and document results. Chapter 3 covers inferential statistical methods in more detail. Designing the research study also requires a population sample of an appropriate size and composition, a subject that is covered in Chapter 4.

SUGGESTED READING

Dietrich FH II, Kearns TJ. *Basic Statistics: An Inferential Approach.* Santa Clara, CA: Dellen Publishing Co.; 1983.

Dixon WJ, Massey FJ. *Introduction to Statistical Analysis.* New York: McGraw-Hill; 1969.

Dowdy S, Wearden S. *Statistics for Research.* New York: John Wiley & Sons; 1983.

Gonick L, Smith W. *The Cartoon Guide to Statistics.* New York: Harper Collins Publishers; 1993.

Huck SW, Cormier WH, Bounds WG. *Reading Statistics and Research.* New York: Harper & Row; 1974.

Ireton-Jones CS. *The Energy Equations: Development of Equations for Estimating Energy Expenditure in Hospitalized Patients.* Denton, TX: Texas Woman's University; 1988. PhD dissertation.

Kazmier LJ, Pohl NF. *Basic Statistics for Business and Economics.* New York: McGraw-Hill; 1984.

Maxwell SE, Delaney HD. *Designing Experiments and Analyzing Data.* Pacific Grove, CA: Brooks/Cole Publishing; 1990.

Stoodley KDC, Lewis T, Stainton CLS. *Applied Statistical Techniques.* New York: John Wiley & Sons; 1980.

CHAPTER 3

Inferential Statistical Testing

James D. Jones

"He uses statistics as a drunken man uses lamp-posts—for support rather than illumination."
Andrew Lang (1844–1912), Scottish author

This chapter covers some of the most common distributions and evaluation methods used in statistical testing. A brief introduction covers the connection between probability concepts and statistics. Important probability distributions (*binomial, normal, student's-t and chi-square*) are described in relation to inferential statistics. The chapter also discusses extensions of these techniques—analysis of variance (ANOVA) and covariance. Finally, regression and correlation analysis, which provide a useful combination of descriptive and inferential techniques, are discussed.

Formulas are presented throughout the chapter for reference, without derivation. The interested reader should consult standard books on probability and statistics for additional detail.

PROBABILITY AND ITS ROLE IN STATISTICS

Probability concerns the likelihood of certain events occurring. An event may be a coin landing with the head up after it is flipped; or it can be a subject on a low cholesterol diet having a final cholesterol level below a given level, say 200 mg/dL. For the coin flip, simple and direct theoretical models govern this event. For the dieting patient, there is no analytical model to predict the outcome; the probability of this event must be estimated by empirical means. Probability theory supplies the analytical support that is used in the more empirical field of statistics.

Probability indicates what proportion of the time a specific outcome of an event occurs. The letter p is used to denote probability. There are many laws of probability. Two laws that are used in this chapter are:

1. $0 \le p \le 1$.
2. If a and b are mutually exclusive events that encompass all possible outcomes (meaning that either a or b must occur, but not both), then $p(a) + p(b) = 1$.

Two functions used in probability for events of all types are the *density function* and the *distribution function*. The density function (also known as the probability mass function) shows the probability of a variable being equal to a given value. It is the theoretical version of the histogram discussed in Chapter 2. The distribution function (also known as the cumulative probability function) shows the probability of a variable being equal to or less than a given value. The distribution function is useful for determining percentile rankings and finding the median.

THE BINOMIAL DISTRIBUTION

Binomial events are those that can assume one of two possible outcomes. Examples of binomial events include a simple coin flip, whether a patient decreases or maintains/increases body weight, or whether serum albumin levels are above or equal/below 40 mg. One of the two outcomes is conventionally defined as a "success." Once the probability of success on a single event is known or estimated, the probability of a given number of successes occurring within a sample population can be calculated. The probability of a success is defined as p; thus the probability of "failure" (the other outcome) is $1 - p$. If N samples are studied in a binomial experiment, the probability of getting exactly k successes is:

$$p(\text{exactly } k \text{ successes}) = \left(\frac{(N!)}{k!(N-k)!} \right) p^k (1-p)^{N-k}$$

The ! sign indicates the factorial function, which is the product of all integers up to and including that number (by definition 0! is equal to 1). The above probability gives the value of the density function at k. To obtain the distribution function, all values of the density function for 0 through k successes are summed.

Example: As the result of experiment or prior experience, the proportion of obese people (those with actual body weight at least 30% above their ideal body weight) in the general population is estimated to be 15%. In a random sample of 10 patients, what is the probability that a given number of the patients are obese? Table 3–1 presents the results obtained using the formula above, when $p = 0.15$ and $N = 10$.

For example, the probability of having 3 obese patients out of 10 is 0.130, while the probability of having 3 or fewer obese patients out of 10 is 0.950.

THE NORMAL DISTRIBUTION

The normal distribution is fundamental in statistics because so many real-world phenomena produce distributions resembling the normal curve. Consequently, many hypothesis tests are derived from normal or closely related distributions. The normal distribution is also known as the Gaussian distribution, named after Carl Friedrich Gauss (1777–1855), a German mathematician and physicist. When considering whether a distribution is normal, a certain amount of judgment is involved. However,

Table 3–1 Probability of Obese Patients in a Sample of 10 Patients

Number of Obese Patients (k)	Probability Density (Probability of Having Exactly k Obese Patients out of 10)	Cumulative Probability (Probability of Having k or Fewer Obese Patients out of 10)
0	0.197	0.197
1	0.347	0.544
2	0.276	0.820
3	0.130	0.950
4	0.040	0.990
5	0.008	0.998
6	0.001	0.999
7	< 0.001	1.000
8	< 0.001	1.000
9	< 0.001	1.000
10	< 0.001	1.000

there are also methods to test the extent of normality in a distribution. A distribution is considered normal if it exhibits the following properties:

- It is *unimodal*, meaning there is only one most common value.
- It is *symmetrical*, meaning that each side is roughly a mirror image of the other.
- It is *bell-shaped* or mound-shaped, meaning it has a rounded middle hump, with tails on both sides that flatten out to zero.

The normal distribution is important because many physical systems conform to the above assumptions. The "fuzzy central limit theorem" states that systems that are affected by many small and independent random factors are normally distributed. A result of the symmetry of a normal distribution is that the mean, median, and mode are all approximately the same value. All parametrical statistical tests assume that the underlying distribution of the variable is normal.

The Standard Normal Function

A normal probability curve is presented in Figure 3–1. It shows the bell shape with the tails tapering to zero with increasing distance from the mean. (Note that this figure uses the symbols μ and σ, standard notation for the mean and standard deviation of a population, instead of the sample mean and sample standard deviation $\overline{X}$ and s. Also note that the x-axis is continuous, meaning it is not divided into discrete values or bins.) With normal distributions, it is convenient to think of how many standard deviations a given point or area is separated from the mean. This is the concept behind the *standard normal distribution*. The standard normal distribution is a shifted, scaled version of a normal distribution having a mean of 0 and a standard deviation of 1. This is a standard way of translating any normal distribution into one whose probabilities are easily expressed (based on number of standard deviations from the mean). To alter the original data from a variable x into a version that is covered by the standard normal distribution, a new variable z is defined:

$$z = \frac{x - \mu}{\sigma}$$

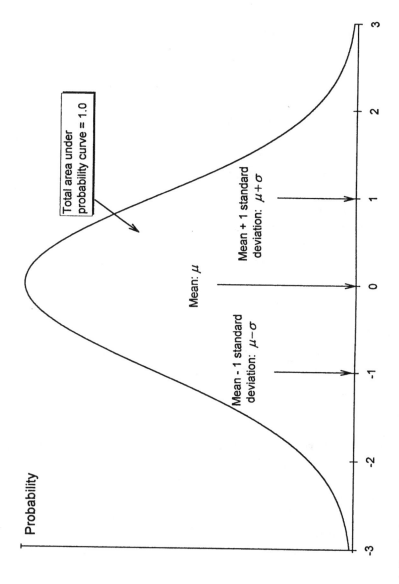

Figure 3–1 Standard normal curve.

Area under the Probability Curve

The area under a section of any density function is the probability of observing a value in that range. The total area under any probability density function is 1. Using the standard normal function, the probability of specific outcomes is easily found in terms of standard deviations from the mean. The standard normal density and distribution functions are $f(z)$ and $F(z)$, respectively, and are plotted in Figure 3–2. (These functions are available in any textbook on probability or statistics and in standard software packages.) To illustrate the concept of area under the curve, the density function in Figure 3–2 is divided into three regions: values less than $\mu - \sigma$ (or $z < -1$), between $\mu - \sigma$ and $\mu + \sigma$ (or $-1 \leq z \leq 1$), and greater than $\mu + \sigma$ (or $z > 1$). Note that the x-axis in these plots denotes the number of standard deviations from the mean. Because the distribution function $F(z)$ is the probability of observing a value less than a given amount, the area in the first region is $F(-1) = 0.16$. By symmetry, the area in the third region is also 0.16. The remaining area in the center region is 0.68. Thus the probability of a value below $\mu - \sigma$ is 0.16, above $\mu + \sigma$ is 0.16, and between $\mu - \sigma$ and $\mu + \sigma$ is 0.68.

Table 3–2 summarizes the probabilities associated with the center region of the standard normal curve out to 3 standard deviations. As expected from the shape of the curve, the area diminishes rapidly with increasing distance from the mean.

Confidence Intervals

The standard normal curve helps illustrate the idea of confidence intervals. A confidence interval is a range of values having a given probability of containing data points of interest. For example, in a normal distribution there is a probability of 0.68 that any given value falls within one standard deviation of the mean. In other words, one can be 68% confident that a randomly chosen data point will be within one standard deviation of the mean. Confidence intervals are commonly used for higher probabilities, such as 0.9, 0.95, or 0.99. For example, the area between $\mu - 1.96\sigma$ and $\mu + 1.96\sigma$ is 0.95; this is the 95% confidence interval. This is also an example of a *two-tailed* statistic, meaning that it measures the probability that the value is either below $\mu - 1.96\sigma$ or above $\mu + 1.96\sigma$. (The small areas

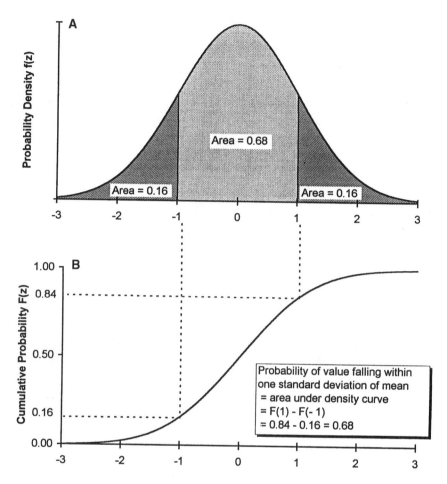

Figure 3–2 Standard normal probability functions. (**A**) Density and (**B**) distribution.

Table 3–2 Probability Ranges of Normal Distributions

Region of Normal Distribution	Proportion of Data Points Falling in This Range
Mean $\pm$ 1 standard deviation ($\mu \pm \sigma$)	0.683
Mean $\pm$ 2 standard deviations ($\mu \pm 2\sigma$)	0.954
Mean $\pm$ 3 standard deviations ($\mu \pm 3\sigma$)	0.997

at either side of a density function are called *tails*.) A *one-tailed statistic* considers only one tail of this distribution and is concerned only, for example, with the probability of the variable being greater than a certain value. Figure 3–3 illustrates the 95% confidence intervals for one-tailed and two-tailed cases.

At this point, some standard terminology needs to be introduced. The term Z_α refers to the *critical value* of z in the standard normal distribution

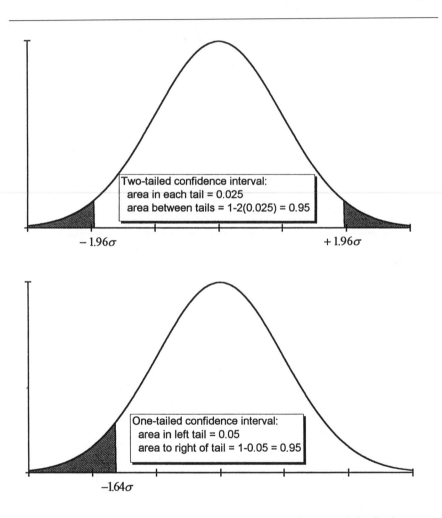

Figure 3–3 Two-tailed and one-tailed confidence intervals for normal distribution.

to the right of which the area under the curve is α (one-tailed statistic). The term $Z_{\alpha/2}$ refers to the critical values of z in the standard normal distribution outside of which the total area under the curve is α (two-tailed statistic).

For reference, Table 3–3 summarizes commonly used values of confidence intervals and the corresponding value of z (the number of standard deviations from the mean) for those intervals. For example, in the two-tailed case, 90% of the probability (area under the curve) is within $\pm$ 1.64σ of the mean and 99% is within $\pm$ 2.58σ of the mean. For the one-tailed case, 90% of the area is to the right of the $\mu - 1.28\sigma$ point (and due to symmetry 90% of the area is to the left of the $\mu + 1.28\sigma$ point).

Example: A group of 73 patients participating in a study of energy expenditure have their respiratory quotients (RQs) measured by indirect calorimetry. RQ is measured as the ratio of the volume of carbon dioxide inspired to the volume of oxygen consumed while the patient is at rest. The RQ depends on many variables such as weight, overall fitness, trauma status, age, and other factors. A histogram of the resulting RQ values is plotted and presented in Figure 3–4. For this data set, the following statistics are derived:

> Mean   = 91.9%
> Median = 91%
> Mode $\approx$ 87.5 – 95% (the histogram bin with the highest count)
> Standard deviation = 11.1%

Because the data are not skewed (mean, median, and mode are all about equal) and generally conform to the requirements of a normal distribution (they are unimodal, roughly symmetric, and mound-shaped), the assumption of a normal distribution here is a sound assumption. This example will be used again later to demonstrate tests of normality.

Table 3–3 Confidence Intervals for Standard Normal Distribution

Confidence Level	Value of $Z_{\alpha/2}$ (Two-Tailed Case)	Value of Z_{α} (One-Tailed Case)
90%	1.64	1.28
95%	1.96	1.64
99%	2.58	2.33

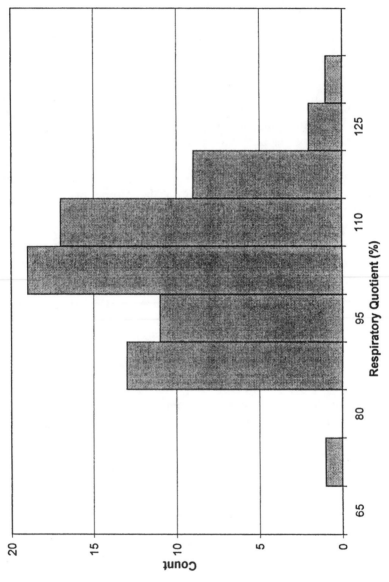

Figure 3–4 Histogram of RQ values of healthy patients. *Source:* Reprinted with permission from Ireton-Jones, C.S.

What is the 95% confidence interval of RQ values? From Table 3–3, the value of $Z_{\alpha/2}$ for a 95% confidence is 1.96. Substituting the values for μ and σ yields an RQ range of 91.9 ± (1.96)(11.1)% = 91.9 ± 21.8%. Thus, the range of RQ values from 70.1 to 113.7% would be expected to contain 95% of the population. For this study, 70 of the 73 patients (96%) had RQ values within this range. (The 95% confidence interval can be used for the general population if the 73 patients are a representative sample of sufficient size. Chapter 4 covers population samples and sample size.)

THE STUDENT'S t-DISTRIBUTION

The Student's *t*-distribution was developed around the turn of the 20th century by William Gosset, who worked for the Guinness Brewery; he was prevented by company policy from publishing articles under his real name and thus chose the pseudonym "student." The *t*-distribution is commonly used for hypothesis testing of small sample sizes (less than 30) when the population being sampled is normal. In practice, *t*-distributions are appropriate when the distribution is unimodal, is symmetric, and has a standard deviation that is not excessive. The *t*-distribution, related test statistics, and terminology are similar to the normal distribution. The *t*-distribution has a wider spread than the standard, normal distribution, reflecting more uncertainty due to the small sample size (meaning it will take more standard deviations to cover a given confidence interval). The *t*-distribution is based on a new statistic, defined as

$$t = \frac{\overline{X} - \mu}{s/\sqrt{n}} = \frac{\overline{X} - \mu}{SE}$$

The *t*-statistic resembles the z value of the standard normal, with $\overline{X}$ substituting for x and the standard error for standard deviation. The *t*-distribution is really a family of distributions that depend on the number of degrees of freedom. The term *degrees of freedom* refers to the number of variables in the sample that are free to vary. The number of degrees of freedom is equal to the total sample size minus one for each statistic that is estimated from the sample.

Figure 3–5 compares the *t*-distributions for two and six degrees of freedom with the normal distribution. For large sample sizes (>30), the *t*-distribution is basically the same as the normal distribution.

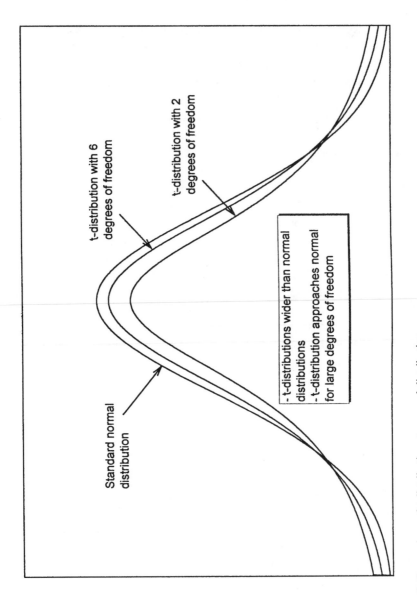

Figure 3–5 Comparison of *t*-distributions to normal distribution.

The *t*-distribution is used for small sample sizes where the distribution is approximately normal. It is used in various situations to test hypotheses of equality of mean values, including the following:

- Inferences about a single population sample:
  1. The *t*-distribution can test the hypothesis that a sample mean equals a specified value by establishing confidence intervals about the sample mean.
  2. The *t*-distribution can test a hypothesis about changes in a sample mean using a *paired t-test* (also called a *matched-pair t-test* or *correlated-samples t-test*). This test compares the same group of subjects or units under two different conditions (such as before and after receiving a given medication or treatment) to detect whether a significant change in mean value occurred.
- Inferences about two population samples: The *t*-distribution can test whether means of two different samples are equal, using a *two-sample t-test* (also called a *group comparison t-test* or *independent samples t-test*). For example, this test could compare whether serum cholesterol levels of two groups of patients are equal. This test requires the variances of the groups to be about equal and uses a composite variance of the two groups, called the *pooled variance*, in computing the value of *t*.

Tests from the *t*-distribution use a critical value of *t*, annotated as $t_{\alpha,n-1}$ to compare with a calculated value of *t*. The critical value $t_{\alpha,n-1}$ is similar to the critical values Z_α or $Z_{\alpha/2}$ from the normal distribution, except that it depends on the degrees of freedom $(n - 1)$ in addition to the significance level (α). Choosing the proper *t*-test requires one to examine the population comparison desired and to adhere to the condition of approximately normal distributions (and possibly a test for equality of variances). Table 3–4 summarizes the applications, conditions, and statistics used for *t*-tests.

Example: This example illustrates the three types of *t*-tests presented in Table 3–4. A dietitian is evaluating a diet-and-exercise program and has measured the weights of the 14 subjects before and after the program. The weight values before and after the program are listed in Table 3–5.

The following three questions can be evaluated by *t*-tests:

Table 3–4 Summary of t-Test Applications

Sampling Situation	Hypothesis	Test Method	Test Statistic and Evaluation Summary
Single sample of one population	Sample mean equals a specified value	Confidence interval (CI) comparison	Calculate critical t value and find confidence interval: $CI = \bar{X} \pm (t_{\alpha,n-1}) SE$, where: $\bar{X}$ = sample mean; $t_{\alpha,n-1}$ = critical value at desired significance; SE = standard error. Accept hypothesis if specified mean value is within CI
Two independent samples of two populations	Means are equal	Two-sample t-test	Calculate t and compare to critical t-value: $$t = \frac{\bar{X}_1 - \bar{X}_2}{\sqrt{S_p^2\left(\frac{1}{n_1} + \frac{1}{n_2}\right)}},$$ where: $\bar{X}_1, \bar{X}_2$ = means of samples 1 and 2; n_1, n_2 = size of samples 1 and 2; S_p^2 = pooled variance $$= \frac{(n_1 - 1)s_1^2 + (n_2 - 1)s_2^2}{n_1 + n_2 - 2}$$ s_1^2, s_2^2 = variances of samples 1 and 2. Accept hypothesis if $-t_{\alpha,n-1} \le t \le t_{\alpha,n-1}$.

Sampling Situation	Hypothesis	Test Method	Test Statistic and Evaluation Summary
Two paired samples of one population	Means are equal	Paired *t*-test	Calculate *t* and compare to critical *t*-value: $$t = \frac{\bar{d}}{S_d / \sqrt{n}}, \text{ where:}$$ $\bar{d}$ = difference between means of samples 1 and 2 S_d = standard deviation of differences between samples 1 and 2 n = number of paired observations Accept hypothesis if $-t_{\alpha, n-1} \leq t \leq t_{\alpha, n-1}$.

Table 3–5 Example Patient Weights before and after Diet- and Exercise-Program

Subject	Starting Weight (lbs)	Final Weight (lbs)	Change in Weight (lbs)
1	126.0	122.8	–3.2
2	119.0	113.0	–6.0
3	151.1	141.8	–9.3
4	133.0	127.5	–5.5
5	148.0	141.8	–6.2
6	158.3	147.3	–11.0
7	127.3	122.3	–5.0
8	136.8	130.3	–6.5
9	155.5	139.5	–16.0
10	148.0	150.0	2.0
11	119.0	113.0	–6.0
12	172.0	165.0	–7.0
13	175.0	163.0	–12.0
14	121.0	121.0	0
Mean Value	142.1	135.6	–6.55
Standard Deviation	18.3	16.3	4.46
Standard Error	4.88	4.36	1.19

Source: Reprinted with permission from Ireton-Jones, C.S.

1. Was the starting weight of the subjects equal to the average weight for adult females? (In other words, if the average weight for adult females in the general population was 134 lbs, is the mean starting weight of the subjects close enough to 134 lbs to consider it to be equal?) This example assumes that a 95% confidence level is desired.
2. Was the starting weight of the subjects equal to the starting weight of subjects from a prior study? (The 18 subjects of the earlier study had a mean starting weight of 130.1 ± 21.1 lbs.)
3. Was the weight loss of the subjects statistically significant?

Question 1 requires a 95% confidence interval using the critical value $t_{\alpha,n-1}$. Because there are 14 subjects (n), there are 13 degrees of freedom

$(n - 1)$. A 95% confidence level sets α at 0.95. The value of $t_{0.95,13}$, obtained from a software package or statistical table, is 2.16. (This compares with the value of $Z_{0.95} = 1.96$ for a normal distribution, meaning that the *t*-distribution is broader than the normal distribution and the confidence intervals are therefore wider.) Using the equations from Table 3–4 for a single sample, the confidence interval (CI) is:

$$CI = \overline{X} \pm (t_{\alpha, n-1})SE = 142.1 \pm (2.16)4.88$$
$$= 142.1 \pm 10.5 \text{ lbs} = 131.6 \text{ to } 152.6 \text{ lbs}$$

Because this CI contains the mean female population weight value of 134 lbs, the starting mean weight of 142.1 lbs is considered to be equal (statistically speaking) to the average weight for adult females.

Question 2 requires a comparison of two independent samples—the two samples of the different studies. The question involves a statistical principle different from that of question 1. Question 1 evaluates whether the starting mean weight of the subjects equals a specific value; it considers the variability of the single sample. Question 2 compares the equality of two sample means; it considers the variability of both samples. Because there are 14 subjects in the first group (n_1) and 18 subjects in the second group (n_2), there are 30 degrees of freedom $(n_1 + n_2 - 2)$. The critical value of $t_{0.95,30}$, obtained from a software package or statistical table, is 2.04. Using the equations in Table 3–4, the pooled variance and *t*-value are calculated as follows:

$$S_P^2 = \frac{(14-1)18.3^2 + (18-1)21.1^2}{14 + 18 - 2} = 397.1 \, (\text{lbs})^2$$

$$t = \frac{142.1 - 130.1}{\sqrt{397.1\left(\frac{1}{14} + \frac{1}{18}\right)}} = 1.69$$

Because the calculated *t*-value of 1.69 is within the range of ± 2.04, the means are considered equal. Notice that the second group mean of 130.1 lbs in this test was considered equal to the first group mean of 142.1 lbs, even though the CI calculated for the first example was 131.6 to 152.6

lbs. This is because the two-sample t-test uses knowledge of the variations in both groups, which causes a larger mean difference to be considered acceptable.

Question 3 requires a paired t-test, because the same subjects are observed before and after the program. This question could be posed in one of two ways:

1. In the first method, the hypothesis would be that the final weights are the *same* as the starting weights. This would involve a two-tailed test to evaluate whether a weight *change* occurred (either positive or negative).
2. The second method would hypothesize that the final weights are *greater than* the starting weights. This would involve a one-tailed test to evaluate whether a weight *decrease* occurred.

The first method would be a stricter test and would require a larger change to be considered significant. For this reason, t-tests most commonly use two-tailed evaluations for mean changes. In either method, the paired t-test compares the starting mean weight of 142.1 lbs to the final mean weight of 135.6 lbs by examining *changes* in weight values, shown in the right column of Table 3–5. The t-test evaluates whether these weight changes conform to a distribution whose true mean is equal to, less than, or greater than zero. Because 12 of the 14 weight changes are negative, one would expect to find the weight change to be significant in either method 1 or 2.

1. The critical value using the two-tailed method is the same as for question 1 above, with 13 degrees of freedom and a significance of 0.95 ($t_{0.95,13} = 2.16$). The t-value is calculated from the equations in Table 3–5:

$$t = \frac{\overline{d}}{s/\sqrt{n}} = \frac{-6.55}{4.46/\sqrt{14}} = -5.50$$

   Because the t-value of -5.50 is less than -2.16, the hypothesis that the mean starting and final weights are equal is rejected, and the weight change is found statistically significant.
2. For the one-tailed method, the same actual t-value is used, but it is compared against the one-tailed critical value of -1.77 rather than

± 2.16. Because the actual *t*-value of –5.50 is less than –1.77, the hypothesis that the mean starting weight is less than the mean final weight is rejected, and the weight loss is found statistically significant.

Regardless of whether method 1 or 2 is used, weight change or loss is statistically *significant*. The researcher must still determine if the weight loss is *meaningful*, given the duration and conditions of the study.

ANALYSIS OF VARIANCE (ANOVA)

The ANOVA is an inferential statistical procedure with the same general purpose as the *t*-test: to compare group means. While the *t*-test compares two group means, ANOVA extends this approach to more than two groups. ANOVA evaluates the sources of variance within a data set, separating the variation due to the individual subjects from the variations between each group. ANOVA is an appropriate technique to use in the following circumstances:

- when more than two different samples are being compared
- when the influence of more than one treatment effect is to be analyzed

The same assumptions are required for an ANOVA test as for the *t*-test: the populations must have approximately a normal distribution with the same variance. The population groups are called *treatment groups* because they often result from a different treatment applied to subjects from the same population. The null hypothesis for an ANOVA test is that all the group means are equal; the alternative hypothesis is that at least two of the group means differ. Rejecting the null hypothesis indicates that a difference is attributable to one or more of the treatments applied to the groups. If the null hypothesis is rejected, further analysis is needed to pinpoint the origin of the differences. A summary of the post-ANOVA test methods is presented later in this chapter.

ANOVA Data Table

The results of an ANOVA test are usually expressed in a table similar to Table 3–6. The intent of the table is to show the variance due to the effect of the treatment, relative to the variance inherent in the population.

Table 3-6 General Format of ANOVA Results Summary

Source of Variance	df	SS	MS	F
Treatments	$k-1$	SST	MST	MST/MSE
Error	$n-k$	SSE	MSE	
Total	$n-1$	SSTO		

In this example, there are k different treatment groups, with a total of n subjects in all groups combined. The groups may each have the same number (balanced) or different numbers (unbalanced) of subjects. Formulas for ANOVA are omitted here, but the individual terms in the table are important to understand.

- *Treatments:* This row evaluates variation between the k treatment groups, a possible source of variation in the means. (Sometimes this row is labeled "between," "between treatments," "between groups," "regression," or a similar description.)
- *Error:* This row evaluates variations in means due to variations in subjects within each treatment group. (Sometimes this row is labeled "within," "within treatments," "within groups," "sampling error," "residuals," or a similar description.)
- *df:* Degrees of freedom for each row. Because there are k treatment groups, there are $k-1$ independent comparisons across group means. Because k means have been estimated, there are $n-k$ independent comparisons within the population groups.
- *SST: Sum-of-squares* for treatments, an intermediate calculation in estimating the variance among treatment groups. "Sum-of-squares" refers to the sum of the squared values of deviations between each sample and its corresponding mean.
- *SSE:* Sum-of-squared errors, an intermediate calculation in estimating the variance across the entire population.
- *SSTO:* Sum-of-squares total (the sum of SST and SSE).
- *MST:* Mean square for the treatments, which is SST divided by the number of df in that row. MST is an estimate of the variance due to the different treatments. Differences between the various treatment groups increase MST, without affecting MSE.

- *MSE:* Mean square for error, which is SSE divided by the number of df in that row. MSE is an estimate of the variance of the total population and does not contain any influence of the different treatments.
- *F:* F is the ratio of MST to MSE, which estimates the variation due to treatment relative to the inherent variation in the data set. Larger values of F show a more significant effect due to the treatments. This statistic has an F-distribution (named for Sir Richard A. Fisher, a pioneer of modern statistics), which is contained in standard statistical tables and software packages. If the value of F is greater than the critical value of F for the specified significance level, the null hypothesis of equal means among groups is rejected; this involves a one-tailed test that indicates an effect caused by one or more of the treatments. The F statistic has three parameters associated with it: the significance level and two different degrees of freedom (one for MST and one for MSE).

There can be many variations in the presentation of ANOVA results. Sometimes the "total" row is omitted and only the first two rows are given. A note is usually attached to the calculated F-value that indicates the corresponding p-value resulting from the test. Sometimes the critical F-value for the chosen significance level is included to show how much the actual F-statistic differs from it.

One-Way ANOVA

The simplest form of ANOVA is the one-way ANOVA, which is said to be one-way because the comparison groups differ from one another in only one dimension—the treatments. A one-way ANOVA evaluates differences among multiple means, given that n subjects are randomly assigned to each of k treatment groups. A different number of subjects may be assigned to each treatment group. For example, a one-way ANOVA might evaluate the differences in the serum albumin levels of treatment groups receiving four different parenteral feeding products. Each patient would be randomly assigned to one of the four parenteral feeding product groups. In this case, the parenteral feeding products form the treatment groups and are the one factor evaluated in the ANOVA. The null hypothesis for a one-way ANOVA is that all treatment group means are equal (indicating no effect of the treatment). The results of a one-way ANOVA are presented in a form similar to Table 3–6.

Randomized Block Design ANOVA

Another form of ANOVA is the randomized block design. This method categorizes or *stratifies* subjects into one of *j* different blocks or groups, based on similar relevant characteristics (for example, age, weight, sex, nutritional status, or disease type). The randomized block design ANOVA resembles the paired *t*-test, except that more than two groups can be examined. This procedure assigns subjects to one of the defined blocks, then randomly assigns each subject within a block to one of the treatment groups. Extending the parenteral feeding example, a randomized block ANOVA might first divide the patients into four blocks: (1) nonmalnourished, nondiseased patients, (2) nonmalnourished, diseased patients, (3) malnourished, nondiseased patients, and (4) malnourished, diseased patients. Then one patient would be selected from each group and assigned to one of the four parenteral feeding product groups (ensuring at least one patient per block/feeding product group combination). Results of a randomized block design ANOVA are presented in a table similar to Table 3–7. This table is similar to Table 3–6 for a one-way ANOVA, except that a row for effect of blocking has been added. The row for blocks includes a term, MSB, for mean-square of blocks; this estimates the variance introduced by the blocking of subjects. This row also contains an *F*-statistic that reveals the significance of the blocking method. It is expected that the *F*-ratio for blocking indicates a significant difference; otherwise, the blocking method is deemed ineffective for revealing differ-

Table 3–7 General Format of Randomized Block Design ANOVA Results Summary

Source of Variance	df	SS	MS	F
Treatments	$k - 1$	SST	MST	MST/MSE
Blocks	$j - 1$	SSB	MSB	MSB/MSE
Error	$(j - 1)(k - 1)$	SSE	MSE	
Total	$n - 1$	SSTO		

ences between the subjects. The null hypotheses for this two-way ANOVA are:

- All treatment group means are equal (indicating no effect of the treatment).
- All block group means are equal (indicating no effect of blocking).

Factorial Design ANOVA

Another ANOVA design is the two-way ANOVA, also known as the factorial design ANOVA. This method tests mean differences among multiple treatment groups for the effect of two treatment factors. This form of ANOVA is said to be two-way because the comparison groups differ from each other in two dimensions—the two treatment factors. A factorial design ANOVA evaluates the individual influences of the treatment factors and interactions between the factors. In the parenteral feeding example, this technique could be used to evaluate the effects of the parenteral feeding product, the method of administering the feeding (such as cyclic versus continuous), and the combined effects of feeding product and method. The two factors in this example are the feeding product and the method of feeding. Performing the factorial design ANOVA requires three F-statistics and three null hypotheses. The null hypotheses are as follows:

1. All the first treatment group means are equal, indicating no effect of the first treatment factor (for example, the parenteral feeding product).
2. All the second treatment group means are equal, indicating no effect of the second treatment factor (for example, the parenteral feeding method).
3. There are no interactions between the two factors (for example, no interaction between the parenteral feeding product and method).

The associated F statistics for these null hypotheses measure the variances due to each of the two treatment factors alone and variance due to combinations of specific treatment factors, all relative to the total population variance. If the third null hypothesis is rejected, the treatment factors are not independent and a relationship exists between them. If this occurs, it affects the interpretation of rejecting either of the first two null hypotheses. For example, suppose in the parenteral feeding test that one combination of feeding product/method shows a significant interaction and the first null hypothesis is also rejected (implying a difference due to feeding product alone). The researcher cannot conclude that a specific feeding product is significantly different, because the test for interaction revealed that the findings may be due to product/method interactions and not due to the product itself.

Results of a factorial design ANOVA are presented in a table similar to Table 3–8. This table presents the variance contributed by each main effect (factors A and B individually) and by the interaction of the effects. This table assumes that factors A and B have a and b different *levels* and that each of the n subjects receives each combination of treatment factors A and B. (For the parenteral feeding example, if there were two feeding products and three feeding methods, then $a = 2$ and $b = 3$.) An actual table usually identifies each factor, instead of referring to factors A and B, and it might label $A \times B$ as "interaction." Factorial ANOVA findings that show significant interactions are often presented in graphs showing the changes in means due to one factor while the other factor is also varied.

Other ANOVA Considerations

Many other ANOVA techniques and variations exist that cannot be covered here. Among the concerns addressed by more advanced ANOVA techniques are the following:

- *The influence of more than two factors.* Factorial ANOVA tests exist to test the influence of more than two factors. In addition to testing the effect of each factor alone, all combinations of interactions

Table 3–8 General Format of Factorial Design ANOVA Results Summary

Source of Variance	df	SS	MS	F
Factor A	$a - 1$	SSA	MSA	MSA/ MSE
Factor B	$b - 1$	SSB	MSB	MSB/ MSE
$A \times B$	$(a - 1)(b - 1)$	SSAB	MSAB	MSAB/ MSE
Error	$ab(n - 1)$	SSE	MSE	
Total	$abn - 1$	SSTO		

between the factors must also be tested. For a test of three different factors (A, B, and C), this means testing for the interaction $A \times B$, $A \times C$, $B \times C$, and $A \times B \times C$. Larger, more complex ANOVA designs rapidly increase the number of treatments and interactions to be tested, and the number of null hypotheses grows quickly. This also results in fewer observations per cell, which can increase the MSE and make the test less sensitive to detecting true differences. Experiments involving larger numbers of factors and levels may result in more combinations than can be sampled. Systematic approaches can be applied to maximize the statistical accuracy when a complete measurement of all combinations is not made.

- *Fixed or random sampling of factor levels.* All the *ANOVA* models discussed thus far are *fixed-effects models* (called Model I ANOVA), meaning that chosen factor levels were included. A *random-effects model* (called Model II ANOVA) includes only a random subset of the different factor levels. A *mixed-effects model* (called Model III ANOVA) includes both fixed and random factors. Random- and mixed-effects models require different techniques because the null hypothesis states that all factor means are equal, not just those that were randomly selected.

- *Repetition of measurements.* A *repeated-measures* ANOVA is an extension of basic ANOVA when multiple measurements are taken on the same subjects. Repeated-measures tests can better pinpoint the effect of a treatment by reducing the "error" terms in variance estimates within the groups. Because repeated-measures ANOVA tests evaluate the same subjects, this method is similar in principle to paired *t*-tests.

Post-ANOVA Comparison Tests

Rejecting the null hypothesis in an ANOVA test does not provide the final conclusions for the researcher. This only demonstrates that a difference exists for one or more of the treatments or blocks that rejected the null hypothesis. Finding the groups with significant mean differences requires a procedure to examine all paired combinations of individual means. Repeated application of paired *t*-tests for this purpose is inappropriate, because the probability of incorrectly rejecting one or more of the many resulting null hypotheses is too high. For example, suppose there were six treatment group means (a, b, c, d, e, f) evaluated in a one-way ANOVA and the null hypothesis of equal means was rejected. To determine which means are different, 15 pairs of individual means (ab, ac, ad, ae, af, bc, bd, be, bf, cd, ce, cf, de, df, ef) must be compared. At a 5% significance level, the probability of finding at least one significant mean difference due to chance alone (by using paired t-tests for all 15 combinations) is greater than 50%. The researcher then cannot resolve a true mean difference from one that occurred due to random data variations. Several methods that adjust for this effect are available for multiple comparison tests following the rejection of the ANOVA null hypothesis. These tests vary in power, or their ability to correctly reject a false null hypothesis. Test methods with higher power (lower probability of type-II error) need a smaller difference in means to reject a null hypothesis but consequently are also more likely to incorrectly reject a true null hypothesis (higher probability of type-I error). Exhibit 3–1 summarizes some common multiple comparison tests used after ANOVA, in decreasing order of power. The choice of which method to use depends on how conservative (lower power) or aggressive (higher power) the researcher wants to be in finding differences between groups.

ANALYSIS OF COVARIANCE

The analysis of covariance is a sophisticated technique that builds on the principles used in ANOVA. The objective of this method is to analyze the sources of variance in an experiment and to adjust for differences in initial conditions that influence the final results. Analysis of covariance compares group means on a dependent variable, after the group means are adjusted for differences between groups on a *covariate* variable. The

---

Exhibit 3–1 Multiple Comparison Tests Listed by Decreasing Power of Test

1. Fisher's least significant differences (LSD) test
2. Duncan's new multiple range test
3. Newman-Keuls test
4. Tukey's honestly significant difference (HSD) test
5. Scheffé's test

covariate is a concurrent measure of the groups that is the basis for the adjustment.

For example, a study may evaluate the effects of two different nutrition regimens on triglyceride levels for two different groups. The triglyceride levels would be measured for groups *A* and *B* before and after applying the nutrition treatment. Suppose the triglyceride levels before the treatment are 180 and 170 mg/dL for groups *A* and *B*, respectively. After the treatment, the levels are 150 (group *A*) and 145 mg/dL (group *B*). The researcher wants to know which treatment decreases the triglyceride levels more (and if it is statistically significant) but cannot simply compare the final results because the group *A* levels started out above those of group *B*. The group *A* levels decreased more than the levels for group *B*, but it is not known if this is a significant difference attributable to the treatment. An adjustment is needed to equalize the effect of different levels before the treatment. In this case, the dependent variable is the triglyceride level after the treatment, and the covariate is the triglyceride level before treatment. The procedure for analysis of covariance is to

1. Adjust the posttreatment means based on the covariate (pretreatment means).
2. Compare the adjusted posttreatment means for significant differences.

Note that the adjustment is made on the dependent variable (posttreatment means) and not the covariate. Analysis of covariance results are presented in a format similar to ANOVA. The table may include the dependent variable both before and after adjustment so the effect of this adjustment is apparent. The discussion should also make clear reference to the covariate so the basis for the adjustment is understood. The statistical significance of results is presented for the adjusted dependent variable. In the example above, the effect of the adjustment may be that the posttreatment means for groups *A* and *B* are 143 and 151 (adjusted from 150 and 145), respectively, and the significance test would be performed on these adjusted values.

NONPARAMETRIC TEST METHODS

The analysis techniques presented thus far have used *parametric statistical tests*, which rely on estimated parameters—typically mean and variance (or standard deviation)—to test hypotheses. *Nonparametric* or *distribution-free* statistical tests can be used when the data do not conform to the conditions required for parametric tests, which include the following:

1. Samples come from normally distributed populations.
2. The variances of different groups must be equal to compare means.

Nonparametric tests are chosen when one or both of the above assumptions are not met. Parametric tests should be used when possible because of their higher power, or ability to detect differences in population samples. Most parametric tests can adapt to situations when the above assumptions are not clearly violated. If the data are clearly skewed, nonnormal, or have different variances, a nonparametric method is appropriate.

Another reason to use nonparametric tests concerns the *measurement scale* of the data. The measurement scale refers to the levels of quantification applied to the data. Measurement scales include the following, listed in order of increasing precision: nominal, ordinal, interval, and ratio scales. A *nominal scale* describes subjects by non-numeric assignments (such as North, South, East, West regions) or arbitrary numeric assignments (such as group 1, group 2, etc.). An *ordinal scale* rank orders subjects by a particular attribute and conveys only that relative rank. For example, patients could be assigned a relative rank (1, 2, 3, etc.) based on their serum cholesterol level. An *interval scale* considers constant differences between measurements as well as rank ordering. For example, the patients could be ranked based on their serum cholesterol level and a score assigned based on relative differences in cholesterol (the difference between 200 and 250 mg/dL being the same as that between 150 and 200 mg/dL). A *ratio scale* expresses a proportion of difference between measured values. On the ratio scale, the difference between patients having cholesterol levels of 200 and 300 mg/dL is the same as for patients having 100 and 150 mg/dL (the ratio is 2 to 3). A ratio scale would not be appropriate for a quantity such as temperature, because the zero point is arbitrary and different results would occur depending on whether Celsius or Fahrenheit scales were used. Parametric tests require the data to be expressed at least at the interval scale. Data measured on the nominal or ordinal scales must be analyzed with nonparametric methods.

There are parametric equivalents to the most common nonparametric methods. These types of procedures have a number of common aspects. Both test a hypothesis to a defined significance level, require a test statistic compared against the critical value, and yield a decision about the hypothesis. Table 3–9 summarizes common nonparametric tests and their parametric equivalents. Details of these test methods can be found in most statistical research textbooks and the more capable statistical software packages. Of the nonparametric test methods, only the chi-square is covered in detail in this chapter.

THE CHI-SQUARE (χ^2) DISTRIBUTION

The chi-square (χ^2) distribution is typically used to compare two sets of data for a "goodness-of-fit" test. The chi-square distribution can be used to compare a sample group to a hypothetical distribution. It can also be used to determine whether two sample groups came from the same distribution. Because the chi-square distribution is a nonparametric technique, an advantage is that sample groups can be compared without assumptions about their underlying distributions.

In principle, the χ^2 statistic measures how much the observed outcomes differ from the expected outcomes. When comparing two unknown populations, an expected or theoretical distribution is synthesized from the statistics of each population, and the deviations from it to each sample group are calculated. To set up a χ^2 test, a number of particular outcomes are defined into k different categories. A category could represent a histogram bin or a specific outcome such as the occurrence of a tail on a coin flip. The number of results falling into each category are counted. The χ^2 statistic is calculated as follows:

$$\chi^2 = \sum_{i=1}^{k} \frac{(y_i - e_i)^2}{e_i}$$

where y_i = observed number of outcomes in i^{th} category, and e_i = expected number of outcomes in i^{th} category.

Calculation of the χ^2 statistic should include only categories for which the expected number of outcomes is at least one. (Some statistical textbooks are more conservative and recommend excluding categories with fewer than five expected outcomes. A reasonable balance is to include

Table 3–9 Summary of Equivalent Parametric and Nonparametric Tests

Parametric Test	Equivalent Nonparametric Test		
	Test Name	Minimum Required Measurement Scale	Summary of Test Procedure
t-test for hypothetical mean comparison or paired t-test	Sign test	Ordinal	Number of values above and below hypothetical median are counted, and probability of observed result calculated from binomial distribution.
	Wilcoxon rank-sum test	Interval	Wilcoxon T statistic ranks data on distance from hypothetical median, sums + /– rank counts, and compares to critical Wilcoxon T value.
t-test for equal means of two independent samples	Mann-Whitney test	Ordinal	All data from both groups are rank ordered, and ranks for either group are summed. Mann-Whitney U statistic tests equality of the group rank sums.
One-way ANOVA	Kruskal-Wallis one-way ANOVA of ranks	Ordinal	The Kruskal-Wallis H statistic is an extension of the Mann-Whitney U statistic for more than two populations.
Pearson product-moment correlation coefficient (r)	Spearman rank-order correlation coefficient	Ordinal	Paired values from two variables (X, Y), each ranked; differences of X and Y ranks are squared and summed into Spearman correlation value r_s or rho.
(No equivalent parametric test)	Chi-square test	Nominal	Occurrence rates of expected outcomes are compared to actual rates; differences are summed and squared into the chi-square statistic.

categories with at least one expected outcome but to ensure that fewer than 30% of the included categories have fewer than five outcomes.) The statistic for a χ^2 hypothesis test also has a number of degrees of freedom associated with it, denoted by the symbol v. The degrees of freedom is calculated as follows:

$$v = k - 1 - r$$

where r = the number of parameters estimated from the sample. Notation for the test statistic is $\chi^2_{\alpha,v}$ where α is the desired significance level. The χ^2 hypothesis test is a one-tailed test, where the null hypothesis is rejected if $\chi^2 \geq \chi^2_{\alpha v}$.

Examples of χ^2 tests include the following:

- *Tests of sample distribution.* A *chi-square goodness-of-fit test* tests the hypothesis that a sample population conforms to a specified distribution.
- *Tests of independence.* A chi-square test of independence tests the hypothesis that the distribution of a variable is independent from another variable.
- *Tests of homogeneity.* A chi-square test of homogeneity tests the hypothesis that the distribution of two sample populations is the same.

Example: A researcher studying a nutrition intervention program of 50 subjects notices that 15 subjects (or 30%) are borderline hypertensive and 5 subjects (or 10%) are hypertensive. The researcher wants to know if this is an excessive proportion of the subjects, which could influence the outcome of the study. For the sake of discussion, assume that prior research has shown that 24% of the general population is borderline hypertensive and 6% is hypertensive (with the remaining 70% having normal blood pressure). Thus, in a group of 50 subjects, one expects an average of 12 to be borderline hypertensive and 3 to be hypertensive. A chi-square goodness-of-fit test is appropriate, because a sample group is being compared to a theoretical distribution. Because there are $k = 3$ categories (normal, borderline hypertensive, and hypertensive) the degrees of freedom are $v = k - 1 = 2$ ($r = 0$, since no additional parameters were estimated). The researcher defines the null hypothesis and alternative hypotheses as follows:

H_0: p (normal blood pressure) $= 0.7$; *and* p (borderline hypertensive) $= 0.24$; *and* p (hypertensive) $= 0.06$.

H_a: p (normal blood pressure) $\neq 0.7$; *or* p (borderline hypertensive) $\neq 0.24$; *or* p (hypertensive) $\neq 0.06$.

Thus, if any of the proportions appear to be significantly other than expected, the null hypothesis will be rejected. A significance level of $\alpha = 0.05$ is specified. The null hypothesis will be rejected if $\chi^2 \geq \chi^2_{0.05,2}$. See Table 3–10 for the components of the χ^2 statistic.

The results of calculations show the following:

$$\chi^2 = 2.80 \text{ and } \chi^2_{0.05,2} = 5.99.$$

Since $\chi^2 < \chi^2_{0.05,2}$, the null hypothesis is accepted and the proportions are not considered out of the ordinary. A software package can also calculate the value of the chi-square distribution for the particular value of χ^2. In this case, the probability is 0.25, so there is about a one-in-four chance of the observed proportions occurring.

Example: The case study presented in the normal distribution section covered a group of 73 patients having the following RQ statistics:

Mean $= 91.9\%$
Standard deviation $= 11.1\%$

Before further analyzing the data, the dietitian may need to know if the data conform to a normal distribution; this information will dictate what follow-up analysis methods may be used. A chi-square goodness-of-fit test quantifies the level of fit to a normal distribution. Figure 3–6 shows a

---

Table 3–10 Calculation of Chi-Square Statistic

	Categories		
Statistic	Normal Blood Pressure	Borderline Hypertensive	Hypertensive
Expected (e_i)	35	12	3
Observed (y_i)	30	15	5
$(y_i - e_i)^2/e_i$	0.71	0.75	1.33

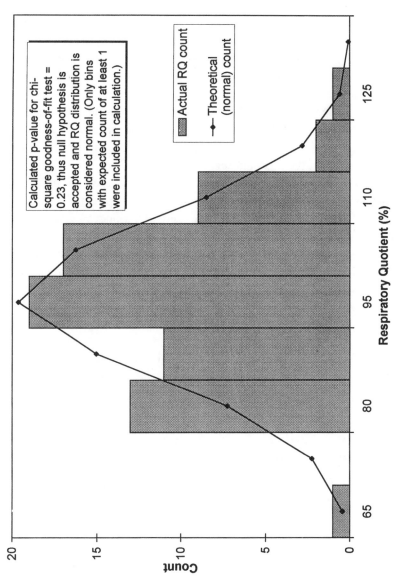

Figure 3–6 Comparison of actual respiratory quotient (RQ) to normal distribution. *Source:* Reprinted with permission from Ireton-Jones, C.S.

histogram of the measured RQ values (in bar graph form) compared to the expected quantities from a normal distribution with a mean of 91.9% and a standard deviation of 11.1% (in line graph form).

The null hypothesis is that these graphs match each other, and a significance level of 0.05 is chosen. For this test, there are 6 degrees of freedom, since the histogram contains 7 bins. (Because the χ^2 statistic is only meaningful when applied to the histogram bins with an expected count of at least 1, the bins for RQ $\leq$ 65 and RQ $\geq$ 125 are excluded.) The critical value is $\chi^2_{0.05,6} = 12.59$; performing the calculations for the data yields an actual value of $\chi^2 = 8.13$. Because $\chi^2 < \chi^2_{0.05,6}$ the null hypothesis is accepted and the assumption of a normal distribution is upheld. (The actual chi-square test for this data set yields $p = 0.23$.)

In the above example the chi-square test upheld the assumption of normally distributed data. Sometimes the assumptions of parametric statistical tests—those of normal distributions and equal variances—are not met. Several actions may be taken if the data are found to violate these assumptions. One such action is to use a *transformation* to rescale the data on a different x-axis. Common transformations used are square root and logarithmic and inverse sine. The appropriate transformation would depend on the shape of the distribution. Another option is to use nonparametric test methods discussed earlier, since these methods do not depend on the nature of the distribution. Another option is to examine the population sample further to determine if the data could be stratified into similar blocks, each of which may be normally distributed. In any event, consulting with a statistician helps ensure that the proper course of action is taken.

ANALYSIS OF PROPORTIONS

Statistical findings of research often are expressed as *proportions*, or the observed probability of specific outcomes. A dietitian may be interested in the proportion of patients who gained, lost, or maintained body weight during a study. By estimating the probability of an outcome as the observed proportion of cases, a researcher can establish confidence intervals and perform hypothesis testing. Table 3–11 summarizes inferential techniques used for population proportions. In these methods, a proportion, denoted by $\bar{p}$, is the number of times a specified outcome occurred

Table 3–11 Summary of Proportions Testing

Situation	Hypothesis	Test Method	Test Statistic and Evaluation Summary
One proportion estimated	Sample proportion ($\bar{p}$) equals a specified value (p)	Confidence interval comparison	Calculate critical z value from normal distribution ($z_{\alpha/2}$) and find confidence interval (CI): $\text{CI} = p \pm (z_{\alpha/2}) \times SE_p$ where: $z_{\alpha/2}$ = critical z value at desired significance (two-tailed) SE_p = standard error of proportion estimate $$= \sqrt{\frac{p(1-p)}{n-1}}$$ Accept hypothesis if sample proportion ($\bar{p}$) is within CI

continues

Table 3–11 continued

Situation	Hypothesis	Test Method	Test Statistic and Evaluation Summary
Two proportions estimated	Sample proportions ($\bar{p}_1$, $\bar{p}_2$) of two different samples (of sample sizes n_1, n_2) are equal	Difference of proportions test	Calculate z statistic and compare to critical z value from normal distribution ($z_{\alpha/2}$): $$z = \frac{|\bar{p}_1 - \bar{p}_2|}{\sqrt{\frac{\bar{p}_c(1-\bar{p}_c)}{n_1}} + \sqrt{\frac{\bar{p}_c(1-\bar{p}_c)}{n_2}}}$$ $\bar{p}_c$ = weighted mean of sample proportions $$= \frac{n_1\bar{p}_1 + n_2\bar{p}_2}{n_1 + n_2}$$ Accept hypothesis if $z < z_{\alpha/2}$.
More than two proportions estimated	Sample proportions conform to a given distribution	Chi-square test	Calculate chi-square statistic χ^2 and critical value of chi-square statistic $\chi^2_{\alpha,v}$ for desired significance level and degrees of freedom. Accept hypothesis if $\chi^2 < \chi^2_{\alpha,v}$

divided by the sample size n. The value of $\bar{p}$ is compared to a hypothetical probability value, denoted by p, or to the proportion of these outcomes observed in a different group. In these tests, the sample size should be large enough to satisfy each of the following constraints:

$$n \geq 30$$

$$np \geq 5$$

$$n(1 - p) \geq 5$$

In addition to the methods given in Table 3–11, the binomial distribution can be used to test a hypothesis about proportions. This can be useful when the above constraints are not met. For example, Table 3–1 listed the probability of obtaining a given number of obese patients out of a sample of 10, given that $p = 0.15$ (that is, given that 15% of the population is obese). If 3 of the 10 patients in a given patient group were obese, then $\bar{p} = (3/10) = 0.3$. The hypothesis to be tested is that $\bar{p} = p$. From Table 3–1, the probability of 3 patients out of 10 being obese is 0.130. If a significance level of 0.05 is chosen, the hypothesis of equal proportions would be accepted because the probability of this result (0.130) is greater than the significance level (0.05). In other words, although there are twice as many obese patients as expected, there is a 13% probability of this occurring due to chance.

Example: A dietitian is studying the effectiveness of nutrition intervention in the improvement of patients' condition. Two groups are studied, with 121 patients in group 1 (with nutrition intervention) and 60 patients in group 2 (without nutrition intervention). During the study, each patient was assessed for improved, maintained, or decreased nutritional status. The results of the study are presented in Table 3–12.

Table 3–12 Nutrition Intervention Study Patient Proportions

Group	Total Number of Patients	Number Improved	Number Maintained	Number Decreased
1 (nutrition intervention)	121	56	9	56
2 (no intervention)	60	13	4	43

Source: Reprinted with permission from Ireton-Jones, C.S.

The dietitian wishes to know if the effects of nutrition intervention were significant in improving nutritional status. A significance level of 0.05 is chosen, so $z_{\alpha/2} = 1.96$. The hypothesis is that the proportion of patients with improved nutritional status is the same between groups 1 and 2; this hypothesis is tested using the difference of proportions method. In this example

$$n_1 = 121, \bar{p}_1 = \frac{56}{121} = 0.463; \text{ and } n_2 = 60, \bar{p}_2 = \frac{13}{60} = 0.217$$

$$\bar{p}_c = \frac{121(0.463) + 60(0.217)}{121 + 60} = \frac{69}{181} = 0.381$$

The z statistic is calculated as follows:

$$z = \frac{|0.463 - 0.217|}{\sqrt{\dfrac{0.381(1 - 0.381)}{121}} + \sqrt{\dfrac{0.381(1 - 0.381)}{60}}} = 3.21$$

Because $z > z_{\alpha/2}$, the hypothesis is rejected and the proportions are considered unequal, indicating an improvement was associated with nutrition intervention.

REGRESSION ANALYSIS

Research frequently yields data suggesting that different variables are related to one another. *Regression* and *correlation analysis* provide techniques for determining the existence and strength of association between variables. Regression analysis was developed near the turn of the 20th century by geneticist Francis Galton, who studied the relationship of heights between fathers and sons. He observed that the sons' heights tended to regress toward the mean of the population, or that tall fathers usually had somewhat shorter sons (and vice versa). Since then, regression analysis has come to mean the development of equations to predict the value of a *dependent variable* based on the value of an *independent variable*. Correlation analysis quantifies the nature and extent of the statistical relationship between the variables. This section only covers *simple linear regression* analysis, in which the relationship between two variables is estimated by a straight line. Techniques for analyzing more than one independent variable and nonlinear relationships are extensions of these methods and are covered in statistical research texts and the more capable statistical software packages.

The following three principal assumptions must be met to apply linear regression techniques:

1. The relationship between the independent variable (the known variable, x) and the dependent variable (the variable to be estimated, y) must be linear.
2. The dependent variable must be continuous, meaning it is not limited to specific discrete values.
3. The distribution of y for a given value of x is normal, and the variance of this distribution does not change as the value of x changes.

Scatter Diagrams

Conformance to these assumptions can usually be determined reasonably well by inspecting a scatter diagram. A scatter diagram graphs individual data points representing an observed pair of values for both x and y. Figure 3–7 presents an example of a scatter diagram. Figure 3–7A shows a plot of a sample set of data that suggests that linear regression is appropriate. Each pair of values (x,y) is plotted without connecting the points. Figure 3–7B shows how the above assumptions can be easily inferred from the scatter diagram. Assumption 1 requires a straight line representation between x and y. Assumption 2 requires the values of y to vary continuously across a range. Assumption 3 requires that y be normally distributed about the regression line with a constant variance for different values of x (this is called the *conditional variance*). All three assumptions are met for this example.

Regression Model

The mathematical model underlying simple linear regression is as follows:

$$y_i = \beta_0 + \beta_1 x_i + \varepsilon_1, \text{ where}$$

x_i, y_i = individual observations of the ith value of x and y

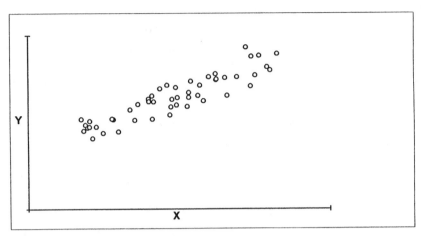

(A) Scatter Diagram of Raw Data Points

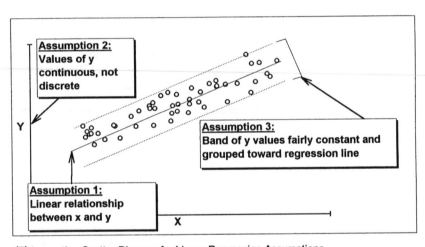

(B) Inspecting Scatter Diagram for Linear Regression Assumptions

Figure 3–7 Example scatter diagram and assumptions for linear regression.

β_0 = y-axis intercept (mean value of y when $x = 0$)
β_1 = slope of regression line
   (Note that β_0 and β_1 are not related to the term β used for type-II error probability.)
ε_i = sampling error associated with ith observation

Figure 3–8 illustrates the interpretation of the β_0, β_1, and ε_i terms. The figure shows that the regression line always passes through the mean values of x and y. The y-intercept, β_0, is shown as the regression line is extended to cross the y-axis. This was done only to show the meaning of β_0. In practice, it is not valid to extend the regression line beyond the range of x and y values used to derive the regression line. The sampling error, ε_i, accounts for the variability in the individual data samples, and differs from point to point.

The line that best fits sample values of x_i and y_i is called the *regression line*. The regression line is determined by a method called *least-squares criterion*, which minimizes the sum of squared deviations between the sample values of y_i and the regression line. The equations are available in statistical textbooks and are built into basic statistics software packages to solve for the regression line given x_i, y_i samples. The form of the regression equation based on sample data is as follows:

$$\hat{Y} = b_0 + b_1 X, \text{ where}$$

X = a given value of the independent variable
$\hat{Y}$ = estimate of dependent variable
b_0, b_1 = estimates of β_0, β_1

The sign of b_1, the slope of the regression line, shows the nature of the relationship between x and y. A *direct relationship* is one in which y increases as x increases, and b_1 is positive (such as shown in Figure 3–8). An *inverse relationship* is one in which y decreases as x increases, and b_1 is negative. Once the regression line is derived based on sample data, a given value of X can be input to the equation to estimate the corresponding value of Y. This practice can be useful in a clinical setting when one variable is easily measured, and it can be used to estimate the value of a dependent variable, provided there is a strong correlation between the dependent and independent variables.

Residual Plots

A type of scatter diagram called a *residual plot* can be used to assess visually how well the regression line fits the data. The residual plot shows

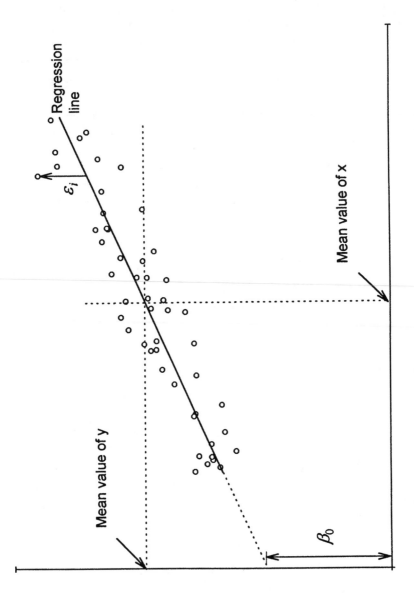

Figure 3–8 Interpretation of linear regression equation terms.

the tendencies of the error in estimating Y. The residual value, e, is the error in the regression estimate for each data point and is defined as follows:

$$e = Y - \hat{Y}$$

The residual plot reveals whether the linear fit is appropriate and if the conditional variance of the dependent variable is constant. Figure 3–9 depicts the residual plot of the data points from the above example; the plot shows that the residuals are centered around 0 with a constant variance, indicating a good regression fit.

Figure 3–10 presents cases where the assumptions of linear regression are not valid. Figure 3–10A and 3–10B show an example where the relationship between x and y is not linear. Figure 3–10A shows the raw data in a scatter plot, and Figure 3–10B shows a plot of the residuals that goes positive, then negative, then positive again. Figures 3–10C and 3–10D show an example of a changing conditional variance. Figure 3–10C shows the raw data in a scatter plot, and Figure 3–10D shows a plot of the residuals that grow with increasing values of y.

Regression analysis can establish confidence intervals for predictions of the dependent variable. This involves confidence intervals for both the mean of the dependent variable and the slope of the regression line. The equations are not presented here, but the effect of this process is shown in Figure 3–11 for the sample data presented in Figure 3–7. Two confidence intervals are shown in Figure 3–11: (1) *the edge of prediction interval*, which is 95% likely to contain all data points; and (2) the *mean confidence interval*, which is 95% likely to contain the true mean of y. The confidence intervals widen as the value of x is further from the mean, because the confidence interval estimates uncertainty in both the mean and slope of the regression line.

CORRELATION ANALYSIS

While regression analysis shows the nature of the relationship between two variables, correlation analysis quantifies both the nature and extent of the relationship. This section covers only *simple correlation analysis*, in which one dependent and one independent variable are compared for

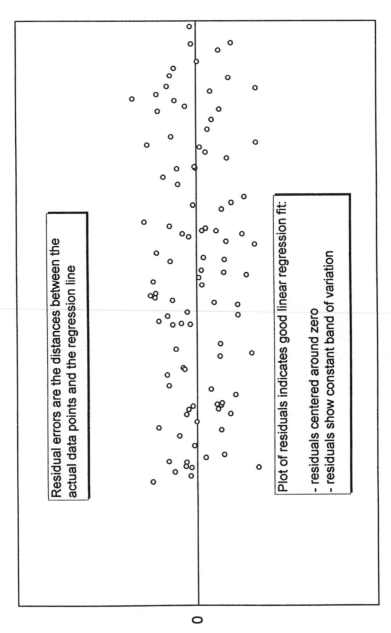

Figure 3–9 Residual errors from linear regression.

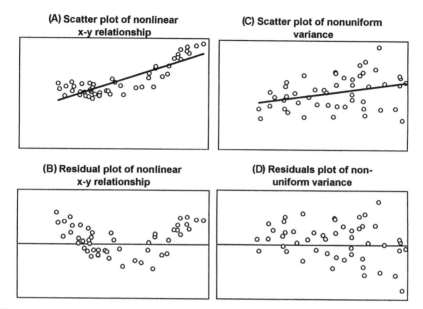

Figure 3–10 Examples of data violating assumptions for linear regression.

association. *Multiple correlation analysis* involves one dependent variable and multiple independent variables, and the underlying theory is an extension of simple correlation techniques. The assumptions in correlation analysis are very similar to those listed earlier for regression analysis.

The fundamental question in correlation analysis is similar to those examined in ANOVA methods. Correlation analysis attempts to allocate sources of variance in the dependent variable. The two sources of variation are:

1. the variation that is attributable to the value of the independent variable (the amount of variance accounted for in regression analysis)
2. the inherent sampling variation within a population (the amount of variance unaccounted for in regression analysis)

The *coefficient of determination* of a sample of values of x and y is denoted by the symbol r^2. The values of r^2 range from 0 to 1, with a value of 0 indicating no correlation and a value of 1 indicating complete correlation. Thus an r^2 of 0 means none of the variation in y is due to the value of x, while an r^2 of 1 means all of the variation in y is due to the value of x.

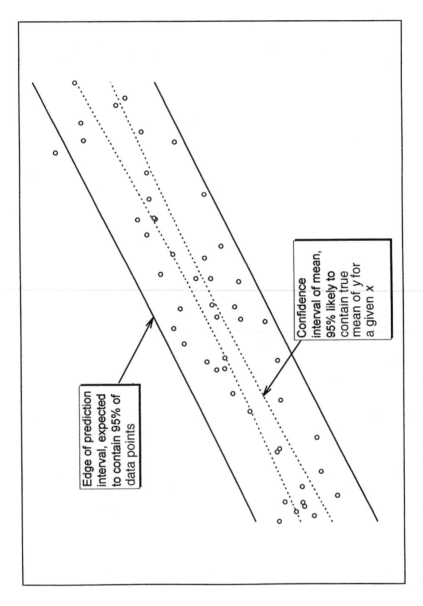

Figure 3–11 Confidence intervals for linear regression.

The *correlation coefficient* (also known as the *Pearson product moment correlation coefficient*) is denoted by the symbol r, the square root of the coefficient of determination. The parameter r is an estimate of the correlation coefficient ρ of the entire population, which was introduced in Chapter 2. The sign of r is the same as the sign of the slope of the regression line, b_1; a positive r indicates a direct relationship and a negative r indicates an inverse relationship. Figure 3–12 illustrates examples of different values of r for various types of data sets. Figure 3–12A shows a strong direct relationship with $r = 0.8$; Figure 3–12B shows a moderate inverse relationship with $r = -0.6$; Figure 3–12C shows a weak inverse relationship with $r = -0.2$; Figure 3–12D shows a data set with no relationship, and $r = 0$. In summary, the sign of r indicates the nature of the relationship (positive for direct, negative for inverse); the magnitude or absolute value of r indicates the extent of the relationship between variables (weak toward 0, strong toward 1).

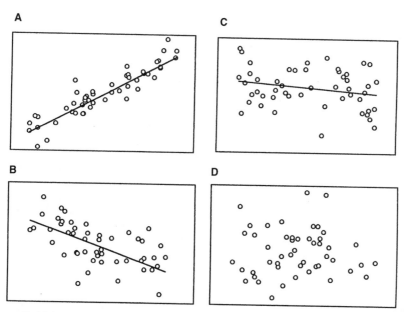

Figure 3–12 Examples of correlation coefficient. (**A**) Strong direct relationship ($r = 0.8$); (**B**) moderate inverse relationship ($r = -0.6$); (**C**) weak inverse relationship ($r = -0.2$); (**D**) No relationship ($r = 0$).

Hypothesis Testing for Regression and Correlation Analysis

Hypothesis testing for regression analysis and correlation analysis examines the null hypothesis that two variables x and y are not related. A summary of hypothesis testing for regression and correlation analysis is presented in Table 3–13. These two methods are equivalent ways of analyzing the same question about whether the variables are related. Either method can be used, and the choice depends simply on which data have already been evaluated.

Example: This example extends the case presented in Chapter 2 for the correlation coefficient between the dependent variable of measured energy expenditure (MEE) and the independent variables of age and weight. That example showed a fairly strong correlation between MEE and age ($r = -0.640$, $r^2 = 0.41$) and a weak correlation between MEE and weight ($r = 0.197$, $r^2 = 0.04$) for the first 12 normal female subjects measured in a study. How significant are these correlations, and how might they change with increased sample size? After collecting data on 33 subjects, the strength of the correlation changed; there was a moderate corre-

Table 3–13 Summary of Hypothesis Testing for Regression and Correlation Analysis

Analysis Type	Null and Alternative Hypotheses	Test Statistic	Test Method
Regression	$H_0: \beta_1 = 0$ $H_a: \beta_1 \neq 0$	$t = (b_1 - \beta_1)\left(\dfrac{s_X}{s_{Y,X}}\right)$ where s_X is the standard deviation of x and $s_{Y,X}$ is the standard error of the residuals	Set $\beta_1 = 0$ and evaluate t against the chosen significance level using the student's t-distribution with $n - 2$ degrees of freedom. Reject null hypothesis if $|t| > t_{\alpha, n-2}$.
Correlation	$H_0: r = 0$ $H_a: r \neq 0$	$t = \dfrac{r}{s_r}$, where $s_r = \sqrt{\dfrac{1-r^2}{n-2}}$.	Evaluate t against the chosen significance level using the student's t-distribution with $n - 2$ degrees of freedom. Reject null hypothesis if $|t| > t_{\alpha, n-2}$.

lation between MEE and both age and weight. Scatter plots of the data for the 33 subjects are presented, along with the residual plots of all 33 subjects in Figure 3–13. The scatter plots suggest a good linear fit, which is reinforced by the residual plots for both age and weight. As the number of samples increases from 12 to 33, the plots suggest an improved correlation between MEE and weight (less scatter) and a somewhat weaker correlation between MEE and age (more scatter).

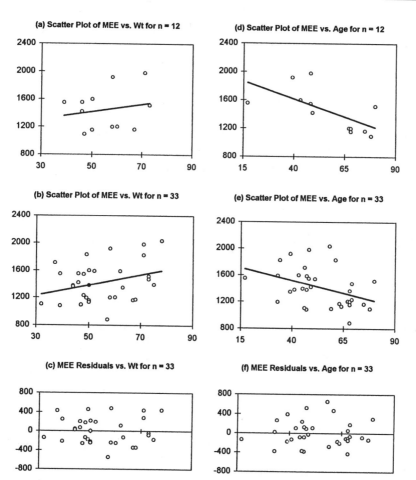

Figure 3–13 Scatter plots and residuals of MEE (kcal/day) versus weight (kg) and age (years). *Source:* Reprinted with permission from Ireton-Jones, C.S.

Table 3–14 summarizes the hypothesis test findings for the first 12 subjects and for all 33 subjects.

Although the relationship between MEE and age was considered significant after the first 12 subjects and after all 33 subjects, the final correlation coefficient was reduced. At the same time, the relationship between MEE and weight strengthened, although the final significance level was above 0.05. (This may suggest the potential for a type-II error—excluding weight as a significant variable when it should be included.) The regression equations after 12 subjects would have caused significant errors in estimating MEE, but the errors are reduced after 33 subjects. Because the MEE shows a dependence on both variables, multiple regression analysis is appropriate to capture the effects of multiple independent variables. Multiple regression analysis extends the concepts of simple regression. Analysis tools for simple or multiple linear regression are included in most statistical software packages.

These data can also be analyzed using ANOVA, which shows the relative contribution of the sources of variance. Table 3–15 presents the ANOVA summary for the relationship between MEE and age and between MEE and weight.

Note that the ANOVA table shows the sources of variance as regression (the variance in MEE explained by knowledge of weight) and residual (the variance in MEE not explained by knowledge of weight). There is one degree of freedom assigned to the regression estimate and the remainder to the residuals. The F-statistic is the ratio of the regression variance

Table 3–14 Effect of Multiple Independent Variables and Sample Size

	MEE-Age Correlation Results			MEE-Weight Correlation Results		
Number of Subjects	Correlation Coefficient (r)	r^2 Value	Significance Level	Correlation Coefficient (r)	r^2 Value	Significance Level
12	−0.640	0.410	0.025	0.197	0.039	0.539
33	−0.390	0.152	0.025	0.319	0.102	0.070

Source: Reprinted with permission from Ireton-Jones, C.S.

Table 3–15 ANOVA of MEE-Weight and MEE-Age Relationships

Source of Variance	df	SS	MS	F	Significance
MEE-age relationship					
Regression	1	409,475	409,475	5.571	$p = 0.025$
Residual	31	2,278,569	73,502		
Total	32	2,688,044			
MEE-weight relationship					
Regression	1	274,143	274,143	3.521	$p = 0.070$
Residual	31	2,413,901	77,868		
Total	32	2,688,044			

to the residual variance (the values in the MS column). The higher the value of F, the more significant the result. In this table, the corresponding significance of the F-statistic is included.

The researcher must use such analysis results to supplement a logical thought process rooted in knowledge of the underlying causes. For instance, based on knowledge of physiology, one would expect that MEE would increase directly with weight and inversely with age. The extent and significance of these tendencies are shown by the statistical results. This may point out the need to investigate other contributing factors as well as the interaction of factors such as weight and age on each other.

The important lessons from this example include the following:

- the value of scatter plots and residuals in evaluating data for linear fit
- presentation and meaning of data in ANOVA format
- the need to understand the physical factors underlying the data

Limitations of Regression and Correlation Analysis

Although regression and correlation analysis are important statistical tools, several limitations or cautions are worth mentioning here.

- Regression analysis is valid only over the range of values measured for the dependent and independent variables. The regression line cannot be extrapolated to values beyond this range.

- A statistically significant correlation does not always indicate a clinically significant or important correlation. For example, in a large sample size, a correlation coefficient of $r = 0.2$ may be statistically different from a value of 0 at a significance of $\alpha = 0.05$. However, the correlation coefficient for this case is $r^2 = 0.04$, meaning that only 4% of the variance in the dependent variable is accounted for by knowledge of the independent variable. (This was the case in the above example relating the dependence of MEE on weight. While weight alone was not a good predictor of MEE, using multiple regression variables—including weight—can improve the prediction of MEE.)
- A significant correlation does not prove a cause-and-effect relationship. It may point to common factors that influence both the dependent and independent variable, rather than a direct causation between dependent and independent variables.

SUMMARY

Probability and statistics provide the mathematical foundation for characterizing and inferring conclusions from research experiments or surveys. A wide range of descriptive and inferential statistical methods is available to assist the researcher in transforming raw data into knowledge. This chapter highlights some of the most important methods, and many others exist and are practiced in research. The choice of statistical methods depends upon the nature of the data, and often certain underlying assumptions must be met to apply certain methods. Statistical analysis is an integral part of many research efforts and must be planned and executed as such. Chapter 4 further discusses the integration of statistical analysis into research projects.

SUGGESTED READING

Cheney CL. Statistical applications. In: *Research—Successful Approaches*. Monsen, ER, ed. Chicago: The American Dietetic Association; 1992:347–372.

Cheney CL, Boushey CJ. Estimating sample size. In: *Research—Successful Approaches*. Monsen ER, ed. Chicago: The American Dietetic Association; 1992:337–346.

Dietrich FH II, Kearns TJ. *Basic Statistics: An Inferential Approach*. Santa Clara, CA: Dellen Publishing Co; 1983.

Dixon WJ, Massey FJ. *Introduction to Statistical Analysis*. New York: McGraw-Hill; 1969.

Dowdy S, Wearden S. *Statistics for Research*. New York: John Wiley & Sons; 1983.

Gonick L, Smith W. *The Cartoon Guide to Statistics*. New York: Harper Collins Publishers; 1993.

Huck SW, Cormier WH, Bounds WG. *Reading Statistics and Research*. New York: Harper & Row, 1974.

Ireton-Jones CS. *The Energy Equations: Development of Equations for Estimating Energy Expenditure in Hospitalized Patients*. Denton, TX: Texas Woman's University; 1988. PhD dissertation.

Johnson NL, Leone FC. *Statistics and Experimental Design*. New York: John Wiley & Sons; 1977.

Kazmier LJ, Pohl NF. *Basic Statistics for Business and Economics*. New York: McGraw-Hill; 1984.

Maxwell SE, Delaney HD. *Designing Experiments and Analyzing Data*. Pacific Grove, CA: Brooks/Cole Publishing; 1990.

Stoodley KDC, Lewis T, Stainton, CLS. *Applied Statistical Techniques*. New York: John Wiley & Sons; 1980.

CHAPTER 4

Conducting and Presenting Statistical Research

James D. Jones

"Like dreams, statistics are a form of wish fulfillment."
Jean Baudrillard (b. 1929), French semiologist

The previous chapters have presented methods used in statistical research. Applying these methods in a study requires a population sample of the appropriate size and composition. This chapter provides guidelines on choosing the population sample to meet the needs of the study. Once the study is under way, graphical analysis of data is a key tool to understanding the outcomes. This chapter illustrates various graphical techniques that help researchers understand the data. Finally, the chapter provides an overview of software packages that can assist in both the graphing and numerical analysis of statistics.

CHOOSING A POPULATION SAMPLE

This section expands the discussion in Chapter 2 of choosing a population sample of the appropriate composition to support the research. Random samples are required in experiments for inferential statistical techniques to be applied. Several sampling methods are listed below.

- *Simple random sample.* A simple random sample is one in which each member of the population is as likely as any other to be chosen, and the selection of one member has no influence on whether another specific member is selected.

- *Systematic sample*. A systematic sample selects subjects on a uniform interval, choosing every k^{th} subject. Systematic sampling is valid if the population members are encountered in random order. This technique is susceptible to any cyclical or periodic nature of the data since every k^{th} member is chosen.
- *Stratified sample*. A stratified sample design divides the population into a number of homogeneous or uniform *strata* based on similar characteristics (such as weight, age, sex, or disease state). A simple random sample is then taken within each stratum. The number of subjects in the strata may differ and, consequently, the proportion of subjects selected from each stratum could differ. For example, in a study on the effectiveness of nutrition regimens on cholesterol, the population could be stratified into five groups based on their initial cholesterol level (Group A: < 150 mg/dL, Group B: 150–200 mg/dL, Group C: 200–225 mg/dL, Group D: 225–250 mg/dL, and Group E: > 250 mg/dL). These groups would be chosen on the basis of expecting the nutrition regimen to have a different effect on each group. The available population may consist of 300 subjects, which result in group A, B, C, D, E sizes of 40, 120, 80, 40, and 20 members. Due to the different sizes, the researcher could use a subset of groups B and C but would need to include all subjects from group E to obtain useful statistics. Differences between block groups could be portrayed in a randomized block design analysis of variance (ANOVA), as discussed in Chapter 3, or similar format if the effects of both the blocking (stratifying) and various treatments are desired.
- *Clustered sample*. A clustered sample design also divides the population into groups, but the membership of a cluster is heterogeneous or diverse. The population is assigned to clusters at the outset, before any sampling is performed. Clustering is typically performed when covering the entire population would involve prohibitive travel or other logistics. For example, patients at four hospitals in different cities may be divided into four clusters—one for each hospital. There is a diversity of elements within each cluster, as patients of various types are cared for at each hospital, but the clusters are similar to one another. Sampling from each cluster depends on the research objectives and composition of the clusters; either random sampling or full sampling of a cluster could be performed.

Ensuring a random sample can be difficult in surveys. It is preferable if the researcher selects the population subjects at random and gathers results from all chosen subjects. The results of voluntary surveys (such as completing an optional questionnaire) should be kept in the context that they apply to the population that chose to respond. The results of such surveys can be meaningful, but their discussion should include a statement about what percentage of the questionnaires were returned.

Control Groups

When selecting a population sampling method, the researcher must consider whether to use a *control group*. A control group is a separate sample of the population that undergoes no treatment and is used as a reference to evaluate the effect of a treatment on another group. The members of the control and treatment groups should be randomly assigned from the same population to allow for a comparison that highlights the effect of the treatment. There are no simple rules on whether to use a control group, but as the number of variables influencing the apparent outcome increases, a control group becomes increasingly useful. Experiments may use either pretest-posttest or posttest-only control group designs. In the pretest-posttest design, variables of interest are measured on both groups at the beginning of the test, the treatment group then undergoes the treatment, and both groups are measured afterward. In the posttest-only design, measurements are made only after treatment.

Blinded Studies

When designing the experiment, the researcher must also consider whether to use *blinded subjects* or *blinded investigators*. Blinded subjects are unaware of whether a treatment being applied is a placebo or the actual treatment. Blinded investigators measure or evaluate groups of subjects without knowing which group has received a treatment. *Double-blinded* experiments use blinded subjects and blinded investigators. Blinded subjects or investigators can be used to avoid introducing bias into the results.

DETERMINING REQUIRED SAMPLE SIZE

Sample size determination is critical because it establishes both the reliability of the statistics and the size of the effort. By setting several key research parameters in the planning phase, the researcher can estimate a reasonable sample size. These parameters include the desired significance level, the nature of the statistics to be compiled, and an estimate of the difference and standard deviation of certain variables.

Initial estimates may indicate a required sample size that is larger than what is practical or beyond the scope or budget of a study. This requires a reassessment of the desired statistical parameters and a recalculation of sample size until a reasonable balance is achieved. In addition, it may be necessary to estimate the rate of subjects dropping out of a study and to increase the planned sample size to compensate for this attrition. It is important to complete such trade-offs at the beginning of the experiment so that proper methods and resources can be applied to the research. In some cases, the sample size is constrained by the available budget or other factors (such as the number of subjects available or the number qualified to enter the study). In such cases, the formulas provided in Table 4–1 can be used to understand how conclusive the statistical research is within these constraints.

The following guidelines can help determine the required sample size to achieve a given accuracy of statistical analysis. Guidelines are given for estimating a population mean or proportion and testing hypotheses about a population mean or proportion. These guidelines do not guarantee that a significant result will be found, because the actual results of a study can differ from the original assumptions. For example, if the standard deviation of a statistic is larger than the assumed value when sample size is calculated, the results may not be as significant as expected.

Required Sample Size in Estimating a Mean with a Given Confidence Interval

The minimum sample size can be determined based on the desired confidence interval and the desired accuracy of the resulting estimate.

Example: A dietitian wants to estimate a 95% confidence interval of the average energy needs of a normal adult patient population and limit the size of that interval to ± 100 kcal/day. The standard deviation of the energy requirements must be provided either from prior data or an estimate (in this case, from a prior study, 370 kcal/day). The value of z for a two-tailed estimate with 95% confidence (from Table 3–3) is 1.96. The

Table 4–1 Summary of Sample Size Formulas

Statistical Test To Be Performed	Statistics Needed To Estimate Sample Size	Sample Size Formula (Round up to Next Whole Number)
Estimating a mean with a given confidence interval	z = critical value for desired confidence level σ = standard deviation of population (or estimate) E = plus-or-minus error allowed in estimating the mean (always one half the total width of the confidence interval)	$n = \left(\dfrac{z\sigma}{E}\right)^2$
Hypothesis testing differences in means	z_0 = critical value for desired significance level (α) z_1 = critical value for desired probability of type-II error (β) σ = standard deviation of population (or estimate) $\mu_1 - \mu_0$ = minimum difference in means that is considered useful (z_0 and z_1 must be of same sign—both positive or both negative)	$n = \dfrac{(z_0 + z_1)^2 \sigma^2}{(\mu_1 - \mu_0)^2}$
Estimating a proportion with a given confidence interval	z = critical value for desired confidence level p = proportion of population (or estimate) E = plus-or-minus error allowed in estimating the proportion (always one half the total width of the confidence interval)	$n = \dfrac{z^2 p(1-p)}{E^2}$

continues

Table 4–1 continued

Statistical Test To Be Performed	Statistics Needed To Estimate Sample Size	Sample Size Formula (Round up to Next Whole Number)
Hypothesis testing differences in proportions	z_0 = critical value for desired significance level (α) z_1 = critical value for desired probability of type-II error (β) p_0 = proportion of population (or estimate) being tested against p_1 = minimum or maximum proportion of population (or estimate) whose difference from p_0 is of interest (z_0 and z_1 must be of same sign—both positive or both negative)	$$n = \left[\frac{z_0\sqrt{p_0(1-p_0)} + z_1\sqrt{p_1(1-p_1)}}{p_1 - p_0} \right]^2$$

value of E is 100 kcal/day. Substituting into the formula from Table 4–1 yields

$$n = \left(\frac{(1.96)(370)}{100}\right)^2 = 52.6 \Rightarrow 53$$

Note that n is usually a fractional value that is always rounded up to the next integer. The difficulty in applying the above formula may be in estimating the standard deviation. In practice, a reasonable estimate of σ may be obtained if the total range of the data is known. In this case, an estimate of σ is one fourth of the total range of variation of the data. In the above example, the data in the prior study ranged from 880 to 2510 kcal/day. One fourth of this range is $(2510 - 880)/4 = 407.5$ kcal/day, which will change the value of n to 64.

Required Sample Size in Hypothesis Testing Differences in Means

This situation presents a method of controlling type-I and type-II errors in hypothesis testing for mean differences by selecting the appropriate sample size. This requires knowledge (or an estimate) of the standard deviation of the population and a minimum difference in means that is of interest.

Example: A dietitian wishes to determine whether the percentage of body fat of a given sample differs from a specified value (or whether two samples differ from each other). Suppose the standard deviation of the population, based on prior studies, is estimated as 9.3%. Suppose also that the acceptable probabilities of type-I and type-II errors are specified as 5% and 10%, respectively, and that a minimum meaningful difference $\mu_1 - \mu_0$ is defined as 3% (so that a "statistically significant" difference is only useful if it exceeds ± 3%). This means that if a true difference in body fat as small as 3% exists, the test is 90% likely to discern the difference, and only 5% likely to declare a difference if it does not actually exist. This is a two-tailed test (since either an increase or decrease is of interest), so z_0 and z_1 are 1.96 and 1.64, respectively (as in Table 3–3). In this case, the null hypothesis would be that there is no significant difference in body fat. The alternative hypothesis would be that there is a significant difference (either positive or negative).

Substituting into the formula from Table 4–1 yields

$$n = \frac{(1.96 + 1.64)^2(0.093)^2}{(0.03)^2} = 125$$

This formula can be used to test whether a sample mean is *different* from some hypothesized value or different from a second population sample mean (in which case the same minimum value of n is needed for each sample). If the dietitian only wants to know if the sample mean of percentage of body fat is *greater* than (or only less than) a specified value (or the first group sample mean is greater than the second), a one-tailed test is appropriate and the values of z_0 and z_1 become 1.64 and 1.28, respectively (from Table 3–3). In this case, the null hypothesis would be that there is no significant difference in body fat. The alternative hypothesis would be that the body fat of the first group is greater than the second group (or greater than a specified value). In this one-tailed example, the resultant sample size n is 82 for each group. It is usually better to use a two-tailed estimate, in the event that the data do not conform to the researcher's expectations.

Example: A dietitian planning a study of albumin level changes in patients who test positive for the human immunodeficiency virus expects the mean albumin level to be about 3.0 g/dL before a treatment and about 3.5 g/dL after treatment. From prior experience, the dietitian knows that the standard deviation of albumin is 1.2 g/dL. The initial study objectives included a significance level (type-I error) of 1% and a power of 95% (type-II error of 5%). Because there is strong evidence that the albumin levels will increase (and not merely change), a one-tailed test is appropriate; z_0 and z_1 are 2.33 and 1.64, respectively (as in Table 3–3). The sample size is calculated as follows:

$$n = \frac{(2.33 + 1.64)^2(1.2)^2}{(3.5 - 3.0)^2} = 91$$

Suppose that due to the budget or patient population, only 50 subjects were available for the study. The next step would be to determine how conclusive the research could be with this sample size. For example, if the type-I and type-II error levels were relaxed to 5% and 10%, the resulting values of z_0 and z_1 would be 1.64 and 1.28, respectively. In that case, the sample size is calculated as 49, so the study objectives can be met with these type-I and type-II error levels and a sample size of 50.

Required Sample Size in Estimating a Proportion with a Given Confidence Interval

The minimum sample size can be determined based on the expected proportions, the desired confidence interval, and the desired accuracy of the resulting estimate. The problem with this formula is that it requires knowledge of the proportion (p)—the very statistic to be investigated. An estimate of p should be obtained from results of a pilot study or other related findings from the literature. (A conservative estimate can be obtained by using a value of $p = 0.5$; however, this could lead to unnecessarily large sample sizes.)

Example: A dietitian wishes to estimate the proportion of patients in a population who have high cholesterol levels (above 200 mg/dL). A 90% confidence level is desired that is to be no wider than ± 0.04, and an estimate for p is 0.15. The value of z for a two-tailed estimate with 90% confidence (from Table 3–3) is 1.64. The value of E is 0.04. Substituting into the formula from Table 4–1 yields

$$n = \frac{(1.64)^2(0.15)(1-0.15)}{(0.04)^2} = 215$$

If a value of $p = 0.5$ is used, the required sample size would be 421. This shows how important it is to estimate a reasonable value of p.

Required Sample Size in Hypothesis Testing for Differences in Proportions

This situation presents a method of controlling both type-I and type-II errors in hypothesis testing for differences in proportions by selecting the appropriate sample size. It requires knowledge (or an estimate) of the proportions of interest and a minimum meaningful difference in proportions.

Example: A dietitian wishes to estimate whether the proportion of patients in a population who have high cholesterol levels (above 200 mg/dL) differs from an assumed proportion of 15%. Suppose that this finding is not meaningful unless the result is greater than 21% ($p_1 = 0.21$), and the acceptable type-I and type-II error probabilities are specified as 5% and 10%, respectively. This is a one-tailed test, so z_0 and z_1 are 1.64 and 1.28, respectively. The null hypothesis is that the proportion is less than or equal to 0.15; the alternative hypothesis is that the proportion is greater than 0.15. Substituting into the formula from Table 4–1 yields

$$n = \left[\frac{1.64\sqrt{0.15(1-0.15)} + 1.28\sqrt{0.21(1-0.21)}}{0.15-0.21} \right]^2 = 341$$

Three other guidelines for sample size apply when estimating population proportions

1. $n \geq 30$
2. $np \geq 5$
3. $n(1-p) \geq 5$

GRAPHING DATA

The display of statistical results can take many forms, depending on the type of data and what the researcher wants to understand from it. A frequent method is to graph the data so they are presented visually. This section presents examples of different types of graphs and situations in which they can be used. Some of the most common types are histograms, scatter diagrams, pie charts, bar graphs, line graphs, and box-and-whiskers plots.

Histograms

As presented in Chapter 2, the histogram portrays how often particular outcomes of an event occur. Values of the x-axis (horizontal axis) denote a particular value of a variable such as patient weight. The value of the y-axis (vertical axis) shows the *relative frequency*, or how often the corresponding x-axis value occurs. The y-axis may be labeled as a count (showing number of total occurrences of each x value) or the relative frequency (showing the proportion or percentage of occurrences of each x value). A histogram can be presented as a *bar chart* or a *line graph* as shown in Figure 4–1A and 4–1B, respectively. When shown as a line graph, a histogram is often called a *frequency polygon*.

Scatter Diagrams

Scatter diagrams are discussed in Chapter 3 as a way of showing the relationship between two variables. A scatter diagram graphs individual data points representing an observed pair of values for both x and y. The grouping of the x and y data points indicates what type (if any) relation-

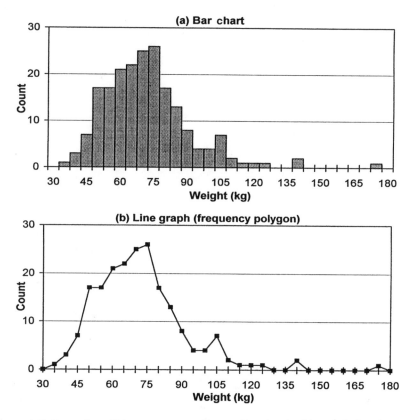

Figure 4–1 Examples of histogram types. *Source:* Reprinted with permission from Ireton-Jones, C.S.

ship exists between the variables and how strong the relationship is. The scatter diagram may also contain a regression line that best fits the data points, along with the equation for the line and the correlation coefficient. Figure 4–2 presents an example of a scatter diagram.

Pie Charts

A pie chart is useful for displaying proportions of a total that are contributed by individual components. The size of each pie slice indicates the

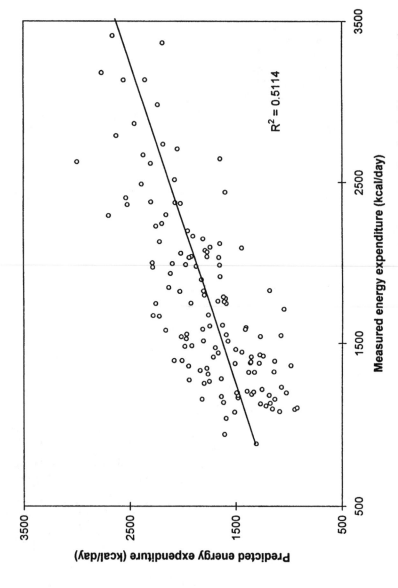

Figure 4–2 Examples of scatter diagram with regression line and *R*-squared value. *Source:* Reprinted with permission from Ireton-Jones, C.S.

percentage of a total that results from that variable. Figure 4–3 presents an example of the food servings in a daily diet that might be recommended from the various levels of the Food Guide Pyramid. The data in a pie chart are typically arranged so that, as one proceeds clockwise (or counterclockwise), the percentage made up from each component steadily decreases (or increases). In this case, the recommended servings are highest for the bread, cereal, rice, and pasta group and decrease steadily through the sweets and oils group.

Bar Graphs

Bar graphs are useful for displaying the amounts of different variables in relation to one another. The length of the bars indicates the value of a variable, and the width of each bar is the same. The variables in a bar graph are arranged in increasing or decreasing order so the difference in values is clear. Bar graphs may be oriented vertically or horizontally as shown in Figure 4–4. This figure uses the same data as in the pie chart of Figure 4–3, but the information is displayed as number of recommended servings per day rather than a percentage of total servings.

Line graphs

Line graphs are similar to scatter diagrams in that they portray a relationship between two variables. The difference is that a line graph connects the individual data points. Line graphs may include *error bars* that show the variability of the data. The *x*-axis often represents time, as shown in Figure 4–5. This figure shows the weights of patients participating in a 6-week weight-loss study. At each weekly interval, three values are shown: the mean weight of the group and the mean ± the standard error of weight within the group. The *standard error of the mean* (SEM) is a measure that includes factors for both variability and sample size. As discussed in Chapter 2, the SEM is the standard deviation divided by the square root of the sample size, and it may be used to establish confidence intervals of the mean. Research articles commonly use SEM values in graphs to show data variability. The error bars in Figure 4–5 are the vertical lines connecting the mean point to the mean ± SEM points. The error bars may be adjusted to represent other quantities such as the mean ± a

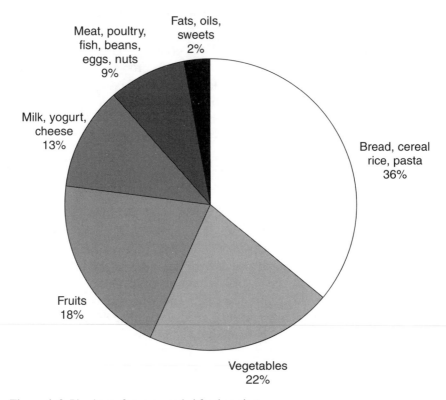

Figure 4–3 Pie chart of recommended food portions.

confidence interval or the mean ± standard deviation. Bar graphs also can use error bars to show the variability of the data in addition to the mean.

Box-and-Whiskers Plots

The box-and-whiskers plot also displays the variability of data. Box-and-whiskers plots may take different forms, such as showing quartiles of the data values. The "box" usually shows some range of typical values, and the "whiskers" extend to the maximum and minimum included data values. Figure 4–6 shows patient weights from four different groups participating in a study. Instead of showing mean ± standard deviation

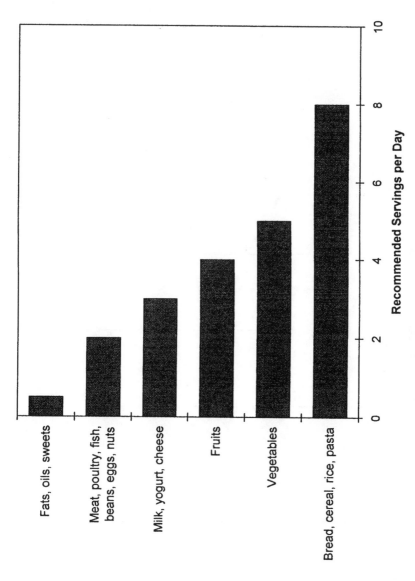

Figure 4–4 Horizontal bar graph of recommended food portions.

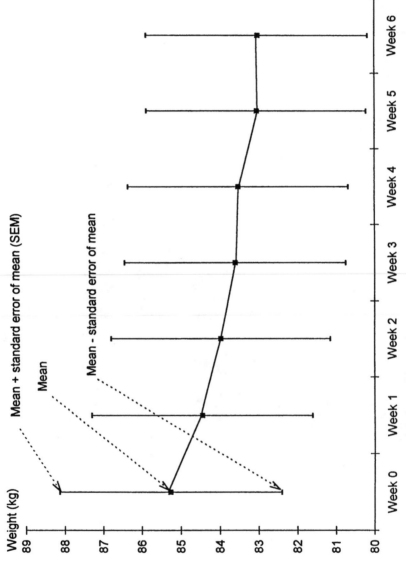

Figure 4–5 Line graph of patient weight loss, with error bars.

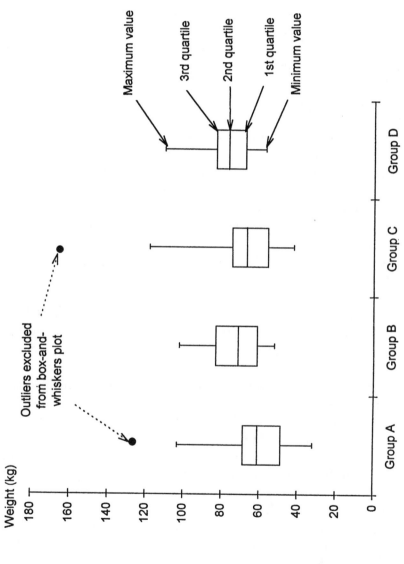

Figure 4–6 Box-and-whiskers plot of patient weights.

ranges, this plot shows the weight value that was exceeded by 0%, 25%, 50%, 75%, and 100% of the subjects in each group; these values are labeled in the plot of Group D as the minimum value, first, second, and third quartiles, and the maximum value. This format allows a visual comparison between data sets that reveals the nature of the distributions of the data. The plots may also show the values of any outliers that were excluded from the box-and-whiskers lines, as in the dots shown above the plots for Groups A, B, and C.

SOFTWARE PACKAGES

Statistical analysis software packages have become more accessible and more powerful with advances in computer hardware and software technology. The choice of what package to use depends on the level of analysis to be performed, the computer and operating system in use (DOS, Windows, Mac, etc.), and the qualifications of the analyst or statistician. Because a software package represents a considerable investment in money and time, the choice should be carefully weighed. This section provides a short overview of statistical software packages currently available. Because the content of these packages can change rapidly, no attempt is made to document the detailed features of the products. The intention is to provide a broad survey of what is available and some items to consider when purchasing software. None of the products listed here are endorsed in any way, but some of the more commonly used packages are mentioned by name.

The first step is deciding what level or depth of statistical analysis is to be performed. This step should include the current and future statistical needs of the researcher, because some of the low-end packages are limiting. This initial step should include a listing of the statistical tests and graphical features desired, the operating system, available computer hardware on which software will be run, and any other applications the statistical software will interact with (for example to import data from a spreadsheet or export it to a graphics package).

Basic statistical calculations are supported by many inexpensive packages (under about $150) or functions that come with popular spreadsheet software such as Microsoft Excel, Borland Quattro Pro, and Lotus 123. These packages can be used to gather, organize, and graph data; in addition, most support common descriptive statistics and inferential tests such as *t*-tests, chi-square tests, simple ANOVA, and linear regression. These packages typically lack more sophisticated functions such as post-analysis of ANOVA results or many nonparametric methods. The graphing features may also be limited. Packages in this range also include add-ons to spreadsheet software that provide more statistical tests or graphing features.

More capable packages begin to fill these limitations, and they typically cost from $150 to $400. In this category, some of the available packages are specialized for medical research, and some fit a particular niche in statistical analysis (such as ANOVA, graphical presentation, or nonparametric testing). As one proceeds toward the high-end (over about $300) statistical packages, many features are added. However, not all of these features are of interest to the nutrition researcher. For this reason, some packages take a modular approach, offering a basic set of features in the entry-level package, with optional add-on packages that can customize the software to the user's needs. For example, some products offer separate add-ons for quality control applications, experimental design, nonlinear regression, advanced ANOVA methods, and nonparametric analysis. Some packages commonly referred to in nutrition literature include BMDP, Datadesk, SAS, SPSS, Statgraphics, Statview, and Systat. These are full-featured packages that support a wide array of statistical methods.

A next step in choosing a statistical software package is to seek the advice of colleagues on what applications they have used. They can provide valuable advice on ease of use, the learning process, and the capabilities and limitations of a product. Among the questions to ask of the vendor are product support (how the user will get questions answered), product upgrade policies, price breaks for government or academic users, multi-user package costs (for networks or mainframe computers), product return policies, and whether on-line user groups exist. Many of the more established vendors have Internet home pages that allow prospective buyers to learn more about the package, to inquire about its features and applications, and even to download a demonstration version of the software.

The use of statistical software is essential in research, and the choice of an application package should be made carefully. The software packages should be chosen to meet the needs of the researcher and should be as easy as possible to learn, use, and expand. The Internet provides a wide range of access to available products and user groups for statistical research appealing to basic and advanced analysts. The key point to remember is that software packages are supposed to be tools that help researchers do their job. As long as these packages have the needed features, are reasonably easy to learn and use, and are cost-effective, they can greatly enhance the work of the researcher.

SUMMARY

Well-planned statistical research can help ensure that the study proceeds in an orderly, efficient, and methodical way. Choosing the appropriate size and type of population sample for study helps ensure data validity with a minimum of time and resources. Many graphical methods are available to reduce and illustrate the data and help observers understand the meaning of the data. Many software packages are available to assist the researcher in reducing and portraying the results.

An important point to remember throughout the research process is the value of each member of the research team. A research project is typically a collaboration of people from different disciplines (including a statistician), each offering unique perspectives to the study. The end product can benefit from that diversity, especially if the research scope and objectives are clearly stated and planned. By applying a methodical approach and seeking the input of all team members, the researcher can achieve the best results that will stand the test of time.

SUGGESTED READING

Cheney CL, Boushey CJ. Estimating sample size. In: *Research—Successful Approaches.* The American Dietetic Association; 1992.

Dixon WJ, Massey FJ. *Introduction to Statistical Analysis.* New York: McGraw-Hill; 1969.

Dowdy S, Wearden S. *Statistics for Research.* New York: John Wiley & Sons; 1983.

Huck SW, Cormier WH, Bounds WG. *Reading Statistics and Research.* New York: Harper & Row; 1974.

Ireton-Jones CS, *The Energy Equations: Development of Equations for Estimating Energy Expenditure in Hospitalized Patients.* Denton, TX: Texas Woman's University; 1988. PhD dissertation.

Johnson NL, Leone FC. *Statistics and Experimental Design*. New York: John Wiley & Sons; 1977.

Kazmier LJ, Pohl NF. *Basic Statistics for Business and Economics*. New York: McGraw-Hill; 1984.

Maxwell SE, Delaney HD. *Designing Experiments and Analyzing Data*. Pacific Grove, CA: Brooks/Cole Publishing; 1990.

Stoodley KDC, Lewis T, Stainton CLS. *Applied Statistical Techniques*. New York: John Wiley & Sons; 1980.

CHAPTER 5

Grantsmanship: Writing and Funding a Clinical Research Proposal

Judith A. Fish and Gordon L. Jensen

Grantsmanship can be a rewarding experience, but it is not an easily acquired skill. Writing a successful research proposal takes training and dedication. The most important aspect of obtaining research funding is experience. This chapter reviews each component of a research proposal and potential funding sources. With a good research question and these guidelines, the new researcher can achieve success.

WHAT IS A RESEARCH PROPOSAL?

The research proposal is the backbone of a research project. In writing a research proposal, the investigator defines the problem and organizes a detailed plan for studying the problem. The proposal also serves as a written document used to obtain funding from an agency, foundation, or industry, and to obtain necessary approval from an institutional review board. After the project is initiated, the proposal serves as a reference source and guide to the research team.[1-3]

THE RESEARCH IDEA

A research project begins with an identified problem or a recognized need. Often researchers recognize ideas through experience and discussions with colleagues or administrators from funding agencies. Ideas should be innovative yet feasible. The most attractive ideas are those that benefit a profession or the public. Inexperienced researchers often choose broad research questions and develop complex proposals that are unrealistic. The best research ideas are narrow and well-defined (see Chapter 1).

After defining an idea, the next step includes reviewing the subject background and investigating institutional resources. A thorough literature search will reveal past research and gaps where further study is needed. Often investigators modify their research ideas, based on others' experience. Learning procedures and potential problems from others can save time and money. Other alterations may be necessary based on institutional demands or limitations.[1,4]

DEVELOPING A TIMETABLE AND RESEARCH TEAM

Once a project idea is well-constructed, a timetable can be developed. This will help in the overall administration of the project and is essential as more individuals become involved. A timetable identifies critical tasks, outlines the sequence of major steps, and determines progress toward the final deadline.

A research team should be carefully selected. Each member (coinvestigator, data manager, data collectors, and statistician) should have a specific contribution and a sincere commitment to the project. Involving members who are overextended or have limited knowledge in the area may only weaken a proposal. A carefully selected research team will contribute to a well-focused research idea and methods. Smaller projects may be better served by consultants rather than a large research team. Seeking advice and input from mentors provides insight into potential issues and concerns; this helps the researcher to avoid major obstacles or pitfalls later in the research process. Finally, every research team needs a principal investigator who makes all final decisions.[5] Although most funding agencies do not state required credentials, most prefer a principal investigator who has a PhD or MD.

FINDING POTENTIAL FUNDING SOURCES

Before writing a formal proposal, it is helpful to have a plan for where the proposal will be submitted. Funding sources vary greatly in their procedures for application. With a focus on where to apply for funding, investigators can better direct their proposal. Table 5–1 lists categories of

Table 5–1 Sources for Grant Funding

Characteristic	Funding Category			
	Government	Private Foundations	Business and Industry	Professional Society or Institution Funds
Available funds	High	Moderate	Varies with the market	Limited
Available application information	Abundant	Often begin with preliminary letter of application	Very limited	Some materials
Funding interest	Wide range but can vary with federal administration	Specific to the foundation	Specific to their products or market	Seed money for novice researchers
Advantages	Secure funding	Fast turnaround time	May not require rigorous review or excessive experience	Fast turnaround and limited competition
Listings	Government publications; on-line services	Professional journals; directory of foundations; on-line services	Not well advertised	Internal publications
Type of research funded	Usually basic science; clinical studies seem to be declining	Varies with the foundation's interest	Clinical trials of products	Pilot studies

funding sources. Each of these categories has advantages and disadvantages. Inexperienced researchers usually seek small, privately funded grants or industry support. As researchers become more experienced in their area of interest, they can compete for larger grants and eventually government funding. Listings of funding sources can be found in libraries and on-line services (see Exhibits 5–1 and 5–2). Industry funding is often not advertised and is usually controlled by the company's research director. For this reason, it is essential for the researcher to build relationships

---

Exhibit 5–1 Funding Agencies

Foundations

- IRIS, Campus Wide Research Services Offices, University of Illinois at Urbana - Champaign, 901 S Mathews Ave, Urbana, IL 61801.
- Sponsored Programs Information Network (SPIN), The Research Foundation of SUNY, PO Box 9, Albany, NY 12201.
- The Foundation Center, 79 Fifth Ave, New York, NY 10003.

Comsearch

- *The Foundation Directory*
- *The Foundation Grants Index*
- *The National Directory for Corporate Giving*
- *The National Guide to Funding in Aging*

Government

- *Catalogue of Federal Domestic Assistance*, Superintendent of Documents, Government Printing Office, Washington, DC 20402.
- *Federal Register*, Superintendent of Documents, Government Printing Office, Washington, DC 20402.
- *NIH Guide for Grants and Contracts*, Office of Grants Inquiries, Room 499, Westwood Building, NIH, Bethesda, MD 20894.
- *National Institute for Occupational Safety and Health*, Center for Disease Control, 255 E. Paces Ferry Rd NE, Room 321, Atlanta, GA 30305.

Source: Reprinted with permission from R. Schiller, J.C. Burge, "How To Write Proposals and Obtain Funding," In: E.R. Monsen (ed), *Research—Successful Approaches*, p. 64, © 1992, American Dietetic Association.

Exhibit 5–2 Online Research Funding Sources

Grant Maker Information
http://fdncenter.org/grantmaker/contents.htm/
Lists private foundations, corporate grant makers, grant-making public charities, and community foundations.

American Cancer Society
http://wuru.cancer.org/grants/egtypes.htm/
Lists research grants for research projects, post-doctoral fellowships, clinical research training, and targeted research projects. Application requirements, funding amounts, and research focus are also included.

Centers for Disease Control and Prevention
http://www.cdc.gov/funding.htm
Lists funding opportunities by subject.

National Institute of Health
http://www.nih.gov/cgi-bin/doc/ind
Lists funding opportunities, eligibility for grants, and application procedures.

American Dietetic Association
http://www.peakcom.com/clinnutr.org/about.htm/
Small grants are available at the national, state, and local dietetic associations. Individual practice groups may also offer small research grants.

A.S.P.E.N.
http://www.peakcom.com/clinnutr.org/about.htm/
Rhoads Research Foundation awards two grants of $25,000 and two smaller grants.

American Society for Clinical Nutrition
http://www.faseb.org/ascn/info.htm

with key industry personnel. Many professional societies have small research funds available to their members. Directories of foundations are available. Most private foundations have very narrow areas of interest. Initial application is usually in the form of a formal letter of inquiry that is subject to foundation staff review. It is important to match a project/proposal to the mission of the funding agency. Most research funds are competitive, but the largest grants are usually only available to researchers with a successful track record.

Each funding source has a key contact person. These individuals should be able to provide information about required format and deadline dates. It is helpful to meet and discuss a project with a funding organization prior to submitting a proposal. If available, proposals from successful candidates can serve as a model for a new proposal.[6–10]

WRITING A RESEARCH PROPOSAL

A proposal begins with a detailed outline containing the key elements of the proposal (see Exhibit 5–3). Sections of the outline can then be delegated to team members. For example, the statistician is most qualified to write the data analysis section. The team leader is usually responsible for delegating, collecting, and combining each section of the outlined proposal.

Exhibit 5–3 Key Elements of a Research Proposal

1. Title
2. Abstract
3. Table of contents
4. Budget and resources
5. Biosketches of investigators
6. Research question
7. Significance and preliminary studies
8. Methods
9. Legal issues
10. References
11. Appendixes

The title and abstract are often the only portions read by initial reviewers or individuals who assign a review committee or study sections. They also are used to stimulate a reviewer's memory when reviewing multiple proposals. For these reasons, the title and abstract require careful preparation and are often written last. The title should reflect the importance of the research project, being both descriptive and concise. The abstract contains the broad objectives and specific aims of the project, followed by a brief description of the research design and method. A good abstract can stand alone as a project summary.

The table of contents usually consists of the main headings of the proposal outline. It may be necessary to include additional sections after the other sections are completed. The table of contents directs the reviewers and research team when they are discussing the project. The proposal writers must carefully follow all page, font, margin, and other format requirements of the funding agency.[11–13]

ADMINISTRATION

The budget for a research proposal may be an obstacle for funding, and budget allowances should be clarified from funding sources prior to submitting a proposal. All reviewers want to feel assured that their money is being used efficiently. A proposed budget should be detailed and complete, and each item should be related to the project and well justified (see Exhibit 5–4). Most funding agencies like to see a commitment from the sponsoring institution. Often a letter from senior administrative personnel of the host institution endorsing the project is included with the proposal. Pilot projects usually attract small grants and should describe plans for future funding from other sources after the pilot phase. Most investigators include a description of the resources available at their institution or shared institutions. It may be attractive to a funding agency to know that computers and technical equipment as well as office and laboratory space are already available.

Most, if not all funding proposals should contain an estimation of direct and indirect costs. Direct expenses are those that are necessary to carry out a research project. These include salaries, fringe benefits, equipment, supplies, travel, and publications. The indirect or overhead expenses are the costs incurred by the institution to provide support services. Examples

Exhibit 5–4 Potential Budget Items

- personnel (including fringe benefits)
- consultants
- computer (and computer supplies)
- equipment
- office supplies
- laboratory supplies
- books and journals
- travel
- honorariums
- telephone, fax, and printing
- postage
- indirect costs
- institutional requirements

include administrative expenses and building operations. The indirect costs are usually a percentage of the total grant and can sometimes be negotiated. Most funding agencies have very specific limits on indirect expenses and award grants only to institutions and not individuals.

The budget not only is for obtaining grants but also serves to control and direct expenses while carrying out a research project. It is not uncommon for a funding agency to expect quarterly reports of expenditures. The budget can serve as the backbone of these reports.

Presenting a well-qualified research team is an essential selling point in a research proposal. This is best presented as a "biosketch" of each key member of the research team. A biosketch should contain information about the team member's education, employment/faculty positions, honors, committees, and publications. As a group, these biosketches should portray relevant experience and qualifications necessary to complete the proposed research project. Some funding agencies have specific forms for biosketches and request a list of other commitments.[1,3,5]

SPECIFIC AIMS AND RATIONALE

Finding a research question should not be difficult. However, finding an important question that can feasibly be studied is a greater challenge.

Young investigators should rely on the experience of a senior scientist to help mentor the development of a good research question. Sources of ideas can come from meetings, journal clubs, new technologies, observing in clinical care, and preparing teaching materials.

For a research question to be worthy of funding, it must be original, ethical, and relevant. It should also require a realistic number of subjects, and the necessary technology, skills, time, and resources must be available to the investigator. Often the scope of a project is too broad, requiring too many measurements on a large group of subjects. It is important for researchers to focus on the main question and avoid unrelated questions.

A research question should be stated in one or two sentences, with a testable hypothesis specifying aims or outcomes. Many projects have several secondary questions. Usually the descriptive questions are listed first and the analytical questions second. All research questions should be followed by a discussion that defines the problem and justifies a research project.

The significance of the research question should be supported by a review of pertinent literature and results of pilot studies. This section should include the most relevant and recently published work. Previous work at the applicant's institution demonstrates experience and success. When little previous work has been done, a needs assessment describing the target population can be substituted. The specific aim of the research project should be related back to current knowledge and how it will benefit patients, advance knowledge, or influence policy.[3,4,13]

METHODS

The methods section requires the majority of time and effort in writing a research proposal. This section should be detailed and based on a sound scientific research design. This section should include an overview of the design and an explanation of how it answers the research question to set the foundation for the more detailed components that follow (see Exhibit 5–5). Sometimes it is useful to discuss other design approaches and why they are not incorporated into the proposal. A diagram may be used to describe a complex design with multiple steps. The study population must be well defined, using predetermined selection and recruitment criteria. Randomization and consent mechanism should be included. It is neces-

Exhibit 5–5 Research Design and Methods

- focused research question
- sound research design
- well-coordinated data collection
- adequate sample size for statistical power
- adequate controls and placebo
- well-designed randomization
- adequate inclusion and exclusion criteria
- adequate variables and measurements
- adequate study period
- appropriate blend
- appropriate statistical analysis

---

sary to demonstrate access to an adequate sample size, and the proposed sample size should be supported by statistical power analysis.

All measured variables require detailed plans for measurement and standardization. All tools and techniques should be justified, well referenced, and related to the specific aims. When alternate methods are available, a discussion should include rationale for the selected approach. An experienced researcher remembers to include methods for quality control and measures used to ensure validity and reliability of data.

The procedures for data collection should be written in a step-by-step fashion. Data collectors, training, and records should be well described. Data confidentiality should also be noted.

Use of a statistical consultant is often necessary and can add credibility to most studies. The statistician recommends data collection techniques, organization of data, and appropriate statistical analyses to test the hypothesis. The statistical analysis section should include power analysis for sample size, and it should relate all collected data back to the research question (see Chapters 2–4).

The methods section is summarized with a work schedule that includes a realistic timeline. Included in this timeline should be development, pretesting, data collection, data review, and dissemination of results. A team organization chart that defines responsibilities and communication lines is useful.

ETHICAL, LEGAL, AND OTHER ISSUES

Every research proposal should include several items to ensure that practices are ethical and that there is agreement among institutions, collaborators, and consultants. A copy of an informed consent form that has been approved by the institutional research review board should verify that participants will be informed of risks and benefits. Issues of safety, privacy, and confidentiality should also be discussed.

Consultants and other subcontracting arrangements can be an added expense, but it is important to justify their value and purpose. All consultants and contracting institutions should provide letters of agreement to participate. A copy of the consultant's curriculum vitae can be included under the appendixes.

References should be included according to style suggested by the funding agency. In many instances, the reviewers are familiar with the field and can recognize errors or misinterpretation of cited references. All references should be double-checked for accuracy.

Technical materials such as forms, letters, previously published work, survey or questionnaire instruments, and data collection tools can be placed in the appendixes.

ELEMENTS OF A QUALITY WRITTEN PROPOSAL

Even a well-designed research project can go unfunded if the written proposal is unclear or sloppy. A proposal requires multiple reviews and revisions before final submission to a funding agency.

The first draft of a proposal should be in a logical order, following the guidelines provided by the funding source. There are often strict page limitations, so it is essential for ideas and concepts to be specific and concise. Unnecessary repetition and excessive verbiage only create a confusing proposal. Above all, every statement should be accurate and well referenced. Each paragraph should be orderly with appropriate format. Logical transitions between paragraphs will guide the reviewer through the proposal.

After the first draft has been revised, it is appropriate to ask colleagues to review the proposal. Different categories of reviewers can provide helpful feedback with different perspectives. First, it is necessary to ask a scientist to review the proposal for design and content. This person should be familiar with the topic. Second, it is beneficial to have a reviewer who has knowledge of the funding agency and past successful proposals. Third, it is helpful to have a statistician review the proposal for its statistical methods and design. Finally, an editor should review the proposal for grammar, punctuation, and spelling errors.

Although it is difficult to receive multiple criticisms, it is far better to receive comments from friends and colleagues than from the funding agency. In some instances, colleagues may have conflicting comments; when this occurs, it is the responsibility of the primary investigator to choose which comments take priority.[1,3,5,13]

COMMON REASONS FOR REJECTION

Most researchers experience rejection of a proposal. The successful researcher has learned to take a failed proposal and revise it for resubmission. Although every review process is different, there are several common pitfalls and reasons for rejection.

Top on this list is an unclear proposal or a proposal that does not follow correct format. When a funding agency has received many competitive proposals, the reviewers reject proposals based on presentation alone.

Reviewers often criticize scientific methods. They may consider some research questions to be insignificant to their area of interest, or too general or overly ambitious. Another potential problem area is the proposal's research design and methods. The reviewers may think that the methods are unsound or lacking sufficient detail. Exhibit 5–5 lists many of the factors that reviewers may criticize on the research design or methods.

Reviewers may also reject a proposal based on concerns regarding the investigator or available resources. Inexperienced or overextended researchers, unidentified key personnel, or a poorly balanced research team are unattractive to a funding agency. The institutional setting may be unfavorable for the proposed design.

Finally, reviewers may criticize the budget or ethical issues. If a budget is unclear, unrealistic, or lacking detail, the reviewer is hesitant to recommend funding. In addition, reviewers may notice a proposal's oversight of ethical issues or unnecessary risk to the research subjects.

Although criticisms and suggestions can seem harsh and difficult to understand, these comments can help the researcher to succeed. The persistent researcher will take all these comments and develop a better proposal for resubmission. Success in research comes with experience and persistence. Because there are no shortcuts in research, success is only achieved with hard work and dedication.[1,3,12,14]

SUMMARY

With shrinking resources and increasing competition, it is necessary to develop a polished proposal. An outstanding proposal requires not only a good research question, study plan, and research personnel, but also a strong presentation. The proposal should be presented in a manner that is clear and concise, with a solid research design. Strong motivation and persistence are required in the successful pursuit of funding.

REFERENCES

1. Orlich DC, Orlich PR. *The Art of Writing Successful R & D Proposals!* Pleasantville, NY: Redgrave Publishing Company; 1977.
2. Twomey PL. Getting started in clinical nutrition research. *Nutr Clin Pract.* 1991;6:175–183.
3. Schiller MR, Burge JC. How to write proposals and obtain funding. In: Monsen ER, ed. *Research—Successful Approaches.* Chicago: American Dietetic Association; 1992:49–69.
4. Cummings SR, Browner WS, Hulley SB, et al. Conceiving the research question. In: Hulley SB, Cummings SR, eds. *Designing Clinical Research.* Baltimore: Williams & Wilkins; 1988:12–17.
5. Cummings SR, Washington AE, Ireland C, Hulley SB, et al. Writing and funding a research proposal. In: Hulley SB, Cummings SR, eds. *Designing Clinical Research.* Baltimore: Williams & Wilkins; 1988:184–196.
6. White VP. *Grants: How To Find Out About Them and What To Do Next.* New York: Plenum Press; 1979.
7. Cuca JM. NIH grant applications for clinical research: Reasons for poor ratings or disapproval of clinical research. *Clin Res.* 1983;31:353–463.
8. *Nutrition Research at the NIH.* Bethesda, MD: National Institutes of Health; 1990. NIH publication 90-2611.

9. Schwartz SM, Friedman ME. *A Guide to NIH Grant Programs*. New York: Oxford University Press; 1992.

10. Schumacher D. *Get Funded: A Practical Guide for Scholars Seeking Research Support from Business*. Fayetteville, AR: Sage Publications; 1992.

11. Reif-Lehrer L. *Grant Application Writer's Handbook*. Boston: Jones & Bartlett Publishers; 1995.

12. *Grantsmanship: Money and How To Get It*. 2nd ed. Chicago: Marquis Academic Media; 1978.

13. Sultz HA, Shewin FS. *Grant Writing for Health Professionals*. Boston: Little, Brown and Company; 1981.

14. Kopple JD. The competitive marketplace for research funding. *J Parenteral and Enteral Nutr*. 1991;15:363–370.

CHAPTER 6

Outcomes Research in Nutrition Support: Background, Methods, and Practical Applications

David Allen August

INTRODUCTION

"The outcomes *movement*,"[1] "the third *revolution* in medical care,"[2] "a technology of *patient experience*,"[3] "a *belief* in the practical superiority of statistical knowledge to other types of knowledge,"[4] "information on outcomes *empowers*."[5] All of these reverential phrases have been used to describe the methods of outcomes research and their application to the study of clinical medicine. Even if one does not "believe" in outcomes research, it is evident that establishment of the federal Agency for Health Care Policy and Research (with an explicit mission of supporting outcomes research), availability of competitive funding earmarked for outcomes research, current emphasis on quality assessment, and the desire of third-party payers to assess and control the costs of medical care ensure that outcomes research will play a prominent role in health care over the next decade.

Outcomes research is certain to affect nutrition care both globally and locally. Globally, the formal methods of outcomes research will be used to design rigorous, often multi-institutional clinical studies to provide data to establish regional and national standards of nutrition care. Locally, outcomes methods will be used by practitioners to refine clinical practice and institutional policies and procedures; they will also be used

Source: Adapted from D.A. August, Outcomes Research, Nutrition Support, and Nutrition Care Practice, *Topics in Clinical Nutrition*, Vol. 10, No. 4, pp. 1–16, © 1995, Aspen Publishers, Inc.

to demonstrate the cost-effectiveness of nutrition care processes and practice within an institution. Nutrition care clinicians must understand both the global and the local impact of outcomes research. This chapter discusses the methods of outcomes research and their application to clinical investigation within the field of nutrition support. It concludes with examples and suggestions to help clinicians apply outcomes research concepts to the local nutrition practice setting.

OUTCOMES RESEARCH

Outcomes research has been defined as "the rigorous determination of what works in medical care and what does not."[4] The purpose of outcomes research is to collect and analyze data to help patients, providers, payers, and administrators make informed choices regarding medical treatment options and health care policy. In both industry and health care, productivity is the relationship between the value of a product and the value of the resources required to produce the product. In both spheres, the inputs are similar; to calculate productivity, one must assign a monetary cost to the value of the input resources. Output in industry and in health care are often qualitatively dissimilar. While it is usually straightforward to assign a monetary value to the output of an industrial process, the outputs (outcomes) of the health care process are often difficult to define and value (see Table 6–1).

By defining and measuring outcomes, one can begin to assess the effect of medical care and health policy choices on the productivity of health care delivery. Outcomes may be categorized as medical, functional, psychosocial, or economic. Specific outcomes may relate to more than one dimension in this array. Outcome variables must be defined so that they can be reproducibly and accurately measured. Outcomes may be assessed in whatever fashion is most relevant (see Table 6–2).

As summarized by Epstein, three important factors have motivated the development of the outcomes movement.[1] First is the concern that efforts directed at cost containment may adversely affect quality of care. Without measures of care outcomes, quality of care is at the mercy of administrative and financial efforts to meet a bottom line. Outcomes must be measured to determine the effects of cost containment on the quality of care. Second, because the concept of competition pervades the health care mar-

Table 6–1 Productivity

Characteristic	Industry	Health Care
Input (I)	Monetary value of the resources required to manufacture a product (eg, the cost of the raw materials, labor, management, and overhead consumed to produce an automobile; the cost of the labor, support services, and overhead to generate a consultant's report)	Monetary value of the resources required to achieve an outcome (eg, the material, personnel, and overhead cost of performing an uncomplicated cholecystectomy; the cost of the personnel, support services, and overhead to complete a nutrition support consultation)
Output (O)	Monetary value of the product (eg, the price of an automobile; the price of 1 hour of a consultant's time)	The value of a medical outcome (eg, the worth of 15 extra months of life resulting from adjuvant chemotherapy for breast cancer; the worth of pain relief afforded by use of epidural narcotics postoperatively)
Productivity	$f(O/I)$	$f(O/I)$

ketplace, purchasers of health care want to know what they are getting for their money. Outcomes measures specify the quantity and quality of the product being purchased. Bailit et al recently reviewed these issues from the private payer's perspective (Bailit and his coauthors are employees of Aetna Health Plans).[6] They noted that management of medical care is the primary value-added service provided by managed care organizations. These organizations ". . . compete based on their ability to control the rate of cost increases and improve the quality of care. In this environment, outcomes research is a critical issue, because the services covered by the plan and the appropriate use of services are primary determinants of medical costs and quality."[6(p AS216)] Third, substantial geographic variations in the use of various medical procedures, even after control for differences in severity of illness, suggest that there may be wasteful consumption of medical resources in high-use areas or suboptimal care in low-use areas.[7,8] Outcomes research can help identify the causes of variations in medical

Table 6–2 Outcomes

Type of Outcome	Examples of Specific Outcome Variables
Medical	Complication rate, mortality rate, weight gain, nitrogen balance, disease-free survival, blood pressure, heart rate after climbing a flight of stairs
Functional	Time until return to work, ability to return to work as a rocket scientist, ability to live independently, stability climbing stairs
Psychosocial	Anxiety level, divorce rate following a surgical procedure, spouse's level of happiness, level of job satisfaction
Economic	Cost of total parenteral nutrition solution used, profitability of creating a home enteral nutrition service, reimbursement for performance of a medical procedure, impact of a marketing campaign on hospital income, cost-benefit ratio of reducing the complication rate of a surgical procedure

practice patterns and resource utilization, and identify opportunities to improve quality of care and/or reduce costs.

Definitions

Because outcomes research exists at an interface between medical, psychosocial, and financial concerns, the terminology of the outcomes movement can be confusing and at times misleading. The term *rationing*, for example, has very different implications and emotional content than the seeming synonym *allocation*. The definitions that follow, compiled and constructed from a number of sources,[9–12] are designed to be practical and to highlight the nuance and significance of the terms listed.

An *outcome* is the measured result of a health care process, system, or episode of care. This definition emphasizes the analytic qualities of outcomes (quantitative and reproducible).

A *standard* defines a set of procedures and practices necessary to deliver acceptable (but not necessarily optimal) care. A *guideline* is a detailed algorithm used to judge the appropriateness of an episode of care. Standards are generally used to evaluate care delivery systems (eg, a clinic, a hospital, a home care agency), whereas guidelines are often used to analyze the treatment of specific patients.

Charge is the dollar amount billed for a service or commodity. *Cost* is the value of the resources (commodities, personnel, and overhead) consumed to produce a given product or outcome. In some circumstances, the definition of cost is expanded to include the personal resources (eg, emotional and familial burden, pain, suffering) associated with a particular set of treatment choices. Clearly, such psychosocial costs are difficult to quantify and compare. *Reimbursement* is the money actually collected for providing an outcome or commodity. Charge, the factor most often relevant to payers, may be quite arbitrary and is often determined by what the market will bear. In contrast, cost relates to the intrinsic value of a service or outcome. Even when analyzing only purely financial costs, overhead items and personnel time may be difficult to quantify. Personal resources consumed to produce an outcome may be even more difficult to analyze.

Three types of benefit analyses are commonly used to assess the utility of outcomes.[9] *Risk-benefit analysis* compares the morbidity, mortality, and reduction in quality of life associated with a treatment to the reduced morbidity and mortality and improvement in quality of life that results from the treatment. This type of analysis is not monetary. While analysis of mortality is usually straightforward, measurement of quality of life and morbidity are often very difficult. *Cost-benefit analysis* relates the monetary costs to the monetary benefits of a health care intervention. This approach may be financially enlightening, but costs may be impossible to determine accurately. Furthermore, cost-benefit analysis has little appeal for clinicians who must deal with patients and human problems that cannot easily be valued monetarily. *Cost-effectiveness analysis* determines the cost of achieving a predetermined outcome. This approach has intuitive appeal to clinicians. To analyze cost-effectiveness, clinicians and patients *a priori* determine the desired outcomes (within the limits of current medical knowledge and technology), and the cost of achieving those outcomes is measured. The most effective intervention is the one that achieves the desired outcomes at the lowest cost.

Outcomes Research in Nutrition Support

Outcomes research is particularly relevant to nutrition support.[12,13] The benefits that result from increasingly sophisticated, costly, and potentially hazardous nutrition interventions must be quantified. These benefits must be defined both clinically and economically. Despite the apparent logic behind the imperative to feed malnourished patients aggressively, aggressive nutrition support (especially parenteral support) is *not* indicated in many instances and may be harmful. The use of routine parenteral nutrition support in critically ill, perioperative, cancer, and terminally ill patients has been repeatedly questioned in clinical trials.[14–16] Outcomes research may provide the methods by which the clinical effectiveness of nutrition support can be demonstrated and its monetary costs determined.

There are compelling professional and economic reasons to apply the techniques of outcomes research to a subspecialty discipline such as nutrition support.[17] Nutrition support clinicians, researchers, and managers have a professional obligation to understand and use outcomes methods and to interpret outcomes research results for the benefit of patients. Managed care now directly affects health care reimbursement for over 50% of the U.S. population.[18] Access to specialty care (including specialized nutrition support) is increasingly controlled by gatekeepers who may not be familiar with the clinical issues faced by nutrition support specialists and who may have administrative and financial disincentives to refer patients for specialty care.[17] Outcomes research may be used to demonstrate the clinical efficacy and cost-effectiveness of specialty nutrition care. Such data are important weapons in the fight to preserve patient access to quality nutrition care and to ensure appropriate professional support and reimbursement for services and expertise provided.

Four user groups may be consumers of outcomes data.[1,17] Patients, third-party payers, nutrition support practitioners, and health care organizations may all benefit from the availability of high-quality outcomes data. All of these groups should have an interest in supporting and participating in outcomes research initiatives (see Exhibit 6–1).

Exhibit 6–1 Potential Consumers of Outcomes Data

- patients
- third-party payers
- nutrition support practitioners
- health care organizations

Patients are the prime beneficiaries of research that defines and improves outcomes. A medical example may be found in the New York State Department of Health program to monitor and improve surgical outcomes in patients undergoing open-heart surgery. Morbidity and mortality from open-heart procedures have been significantly reduced as a result of a statewide effort that collects data on all patients and their treatment and uses these data to inform clinicians, hospitals, and the public.[19,20] Quality of life may also be improved through the use of outcomes research methods. In an influential study published in 1992, the Nordic Gastrointestinal Tumor Adjuvant Therapy Group investigated whether early chemotherapy in asymptomatic patients with advanced colorectal cancer improved the length of survival and the length of symptom-free survival in comparison to chemotherapy delayed until the onset of symptoms. They found that early initiation of chemotherapy, despite its potential toxicity in asymptomatic patients, prolonged symptom-free survival and thereby improved quality of life. The study was informative only because the researchers specifically chose to look at quality of life as an outcome.[21]

Third-party payers can benefit significantly from the availability of good outcomes data. Cost-effective management of patient outcomes is the service that generates profits for insurers. Payers require quality data on outcomes to assess the quality and cost of care. With this knowledge, third-party payers can more effectively manage care, and consequently achieve better profit margins. Managed care organizations are particularly interested in information concerning technologies, procedures, and care plans that have a significant impact on improving health and/or increasing the efficiency of care. They are often more interested in the applicability of the data than its rigor or biologic significance.[6]

Nutrition support practitioners should be avid consumers of outcomes information. Beyond a personal and professional interest in good outcomes for patients, outcomes data are becoming increasingly important in the defense of funding for specialty nutrition care and for nutrition support teams. In an era of "downsizing," professional and personal job security is increasingly dependent upon demonstrating that nutrition care providers' clinical and administrative activities reduce morbidity and mortality, decrease lengths of stay, reduce costs of care, and improve functional and psychosocial outcomes.

Health care organizations (hospitals, long-term care facilities, home care organizations, etc) must also increasingly depend upon outcomes data to improve the ways they do business. Financial pressures are forcing these organizations to do more with less. Clinical pathways validated with data obtained from outcomes studies are one tool that can be used to improve the quality and cost-effectiveness of care processes.[22,23] Resultant better outcomes may be used to seek increased reimbursement for specialty services such as nutrition support while simultaneously reducing institutional costs.

OUTCOMES RESEARCH METHODS

Outcomes research is based upon the premise that analysis of the outcomes of medical care can identify factors that may be altered to improve subsequent outcomes.[24–28] Conceptually, variations in outcomes may be attributed to quality of care, severity of illness, the presence of comorbidities, demographic factors, and randomness (see Figure 6-1).[27,29]

Severity of illness, the presence of comorbidities, demographics, and randomness are uncontrollable aspects of medical care. They cannot be easily altered with currently available technology and knowledge. Quality of care embodies the controllable factors—that is, the facilities, personnel, infra-

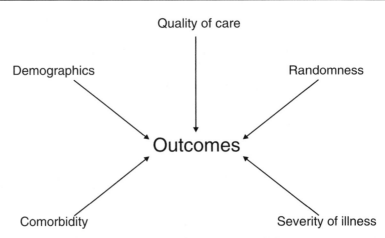

Figure 6–1 Factors causing variations in health care outcomes. Variations in outcomes may be attributed to quality of care, severity of illness, the presence of comorbidities, demographic factors, and randomness. Quality of care embodies those controllable factors that may be manipulated to improve outcomes.

structure, technology, knowledge base, decision making, technical capabilities, and care processes (eg, care algorithms, clinical pathways, quality assurance programs)—that influence patient outcomes and that can be engineered in ways that improve those outcomes.

Outcomes research assumes that adverse outcomes are markers for bad care.[19,24–31] Outcomes research methods are designed to adjust for the uncontrollable factors listed above and thereby highlight the influence of controllable factors (quality of care) on the quality of outcomes. When the influence of quality of care on outcomes is understood, interventions may be undertaken to improve outcomes. These interventions should change controllable elements of care to improve the quality of care.

Consider the following example. Hospital B has lower morbidity and mortality rates (better outcomes) than Hospital A for patients undergoing pancreaticoduodenectomy (Whipple procedure). Analysis demonstrates that patients operated on at Hospital A are older (demographics), have a higher incidence of ischemic heart disease (comorbidity), and have larger pancreatic cancers (severity of illness) than those patients operated on at Hospital B. The uncontrollable factors at Hospital A suggest that the patients seen at that institution are inherently less likely to have good outcomes. When the uncontrollable factors are adjusted for, it becomes apparent that patients at Hospital A actually have better outcomes than *comparable* patients operated on at Hospital B. Further investigation suggests that much of the relatively increased morbidity and mortality observed at Hospital B is attributable to two surgeons who perform few pancreaticoduodenectomies. Quality of care may be improved, with resultant improved outcomes, by interventions targeted at improving the care provided by the two less-experienced surgeons (perhaps by requiring them to operate with a more-experienced colleague as the first assistant).

The focus of outcomes research is the improvement of patient care by improving the quality of care. To study the impact of quality of care on outcomes, one must control for the influences of severity of illness, demographics, and comorbidity, and statistically understand the possible confounding variation that results from randomness.

It is especially difficult to understand the impact of quality of nutrition care upon patient outcomes. Because nutrition support is almost always adjunctive, one can expect the portion of outcomes that is attributable to the quality of the nutrition care to be small. Therefore, even large changes in nutrition care may be only minimally evident when outcomes are analyzed. Nutrition support has only a marginal effect on outcomes because outcomes are dominated by severity of illness, comorbidity, patient demographics, and disease-specific therapies. Accurate outcomes assessment and large numbers of patients are required to detect the small (but probably significant) effect of nutrition support.[32–34]

Conceptual Approach

The assessment of quality of care and cost-effectiveness of care can be modeled as a five-step process (see Figure 6–2).[29] The first step involves establishment of a risk-adjusted model for outcomes. This entails the use of expert judgment and clinical experience to define the relevant outcomes measures (eg, mortality, return to work, depression index, weight gain) and to specify candidate risk factors (factors that are present before

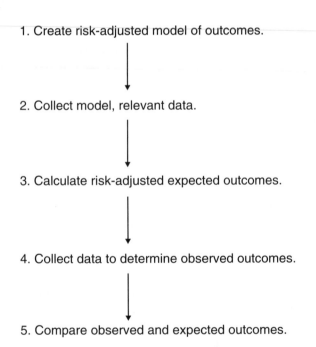

Figure 6–2 Five-step process in assessment of quality and cost-effectiveness of care.

the care being studied is initiated) that are likely to have a significant influence on the outcomes. The outcomes are dependent variables (dependent upon the risk factors that must be adjusted for and dependent upon the process being studied), and the risk factors are independent variables.

The second step requires collection of model, relevant data. In this step, a standard population is chosen that should share many of the attributes of the patient population in whom outcomes will ultimately be studied. Outcomes and risk factor information are collected in the standard population. During this step, much can be learned about the availability and reliability of data collection; the knowledge gained should be used to modify data collection methods and simplify subsequent efforts.

In the third step, data collected in the standard population are used to calculate expected outcomes for patients with various mixes of risk factors. This involves creation of a mathematical model that relates patient outcomes to the presence, absence, and magnitude of risk factors. In the mathematical model, it is likely that many of the factors originally proposed in the expert risk-adjusted model will prove not to be useful (they will not turn out to be statistically significant predictors of outcomes). A variety of statistical methods are available to allow prediction of expected outcomes from an experience-based database that contains information about outcomes and risk factors.[29,31,35]

Fourth, information about outcomes, risk factors, and quality of care is collected in the patient population of interest. This is the data set that will be used to perform the formal outcomes analysis.

In the fifth and final step, the outcomes observed in the population of interest are compared to the outcomes that are expected in that patient group. The expected outcomes are calculated by using the risk factors observed in the population of interest as the independent variables in the mathematical model generated in step 3. Comparison of expected and observed outcomes identifies areas where outcomes were either better or worse than expected. Because the expected outcomes are risk adjusted, the observed differences should be attributable to differences in quality of care. Data concerning the controllable quality-of-care factors are then analyzed (generally using multivariate techniques) to identify opportunities to improve outcomes and to highlight especially high-quality care.

To simplify this process, risk adjustment for severity of illness, comorbidity, and demographic factors can often be reliably accomplished using a small set of readily available data elements.[25-30,32-34,36] From these available models, expected risk of death, complications, and readmission may be computed.[32-34,37,38]

Methodology

For the multivariate statistical methods generally applied to analysis of outcomes data sets to perform well, the number of "events" (deaths, complications, or other undesirable outcomes) should exceed the number of risk factors by a factor of at least 10.[31,35,39,40] For example, to analyze the influences on an adverse outcome that occurs an average of 5% of the time and that the risk model suggests is influenced by 10 risk factors, at least 2000 patients at risk for the adverse outcome must be incorporated into the database (in 2000 patients, 100 adverse events would be expected, 10 times the number of risk factors in the model). In practice, larger numbers of patients are required to allow for incomplete or inaccurate data collection, and because more than one outcome is usually assessed simultaneously.

Access to tens of thousands of patients generally requires a multi-institutional, cooperative effort. This places a premium on reliable, accurate, standardized, complete, and cost-effective data collection. Although retrospective data collection is possible,[40] most large efforts of this type that use data elements beyond those available in administrative databases (generally hospital and insurer based) have focused on prospective data acquisition.[19,31] In addition, such efforts invest substantially in definition of data elements; development of shared hardware, software, and network resources to facilitate data collection, transmission, and analysis; and creation of quality assurance mechanisms (eg, site visits, data manager training, data verification, methodology and results reporting workshops).[19,31]

Four other methodologic issues are worth mentioning within the context of large-scale outcomes studies, although they are equally pertinent to small-scale projects.

1. choice of outcomes measures
2. use of intermediate end points
3. measurement of costs
4. sensitivity analysis

Choice of Outcomes Measures

The choice of outcomes measures is crucial to the design and evaluation of outcomes studies (see Table 6–3). The outcomes end points must be objective, precise, quantitative, and translatable to multiple institutions. Some outcomes are easy to measure (eg, death, presence of pneumothorax, ability to walk). Other outcomes (such as anxiety level, state of well-being, and opportunity cost of being out of work) may be equally important but quite difficult to measure. Generally, outcomes measures should be chosen so that they can be reliably and reproducibly measured, so they are relevant and interesting to experts in the field, and so demonstrated differences are clinically and statistically significant (a difference, to be a difference, must make a difference).

Table 6–3 Attributes of Good Outcome Variables

Attribute	Well-Defined Variable	Poorly Defined Variable
Objective	Anxiety level measured using validated multi-item assessment questionnaire.	Clinician elicits patient assessment of personal anxiety level in an unstructured interview.
Precise	Nutrition status assessed using defined elements of the history, physical exam, and laboratory data to classify patients into one of four categories.	Nutrition status assessed by clinicians subjectively as either malnourished or well nourished.
Quantitative	Tumor response to therapy assessed from the product of bidirectional measurements of the size of the largest pulmonary metastasis on a chest CT scan.	Tumor response to therapy assessed by reviewing medical record progress notes written by patients' primary clinicians.
Translatable	Clinical laboratory costs assessed by assigning a relative value to each laboratory study performed and then summing the relative value costs for each patient at each study site.	Clinical laboratory costs assessed by reviewing hospital financial data and adding up the clinical laboratory charges for each patient at each study site.

Use of Intermediate End Points

Ideally, all patients in an outcomes database should be followed until they are no longer at risk for an adverse outcome. In practice, it may be prohibitively complex and expensive to follow patients until all end points (eg, death, return to work, effect of illness on spousal relationships) have been observed. Often, surrogate (intermediate) end points must be chosen to substitute for the actual outcomes of interest. For example, instead of following patients until they return to work, an occupational medicine assessment at the time of hospital discharge may suffice to predict accurately the time until return to work. Use of surrogate end points may be very cost-effective, but the end points must be validated to demonstrate that they accurately predict the outcome of interest.

Measurement of Costs

Cost, the actual value of resources consumed to achieve a specified outcome, is difficult to measure. It is difficult to compare costs between study sites. Costs should not be confused with charges or with collections. It is beyond the scope of this chapter to discuss actual approaches to analysis of costs. During study design and interpretation, researchers must carefully consider these issues.

Sensitivity Analysis

All outcomes studies require estimation or measurement of parameters such as cost, impact of interventions on length of hospitalization, and proportion of complications prevented by a treatment. If the conclusions of a study are critically dependent on the value of a particular estimated or measured parameter, the study results are referred to as being *sensitive* to the choice of the value of the parameter. A hypothetical example is shown in Figure 6–3, which illustrates the cumulative cost of complications resulting from a surgical procedure. If an intervention (such as nutrition support) decreases the usual complication rate from 40% to 20%, the cost savings will be related to the cost per complication, which corresponds to the slopes of lines A and B. If the cost per complication is estimated or measured to be low (line B), the cost savings resulting from the intervention will be relatively small (ΔB); if the cost savings per complication avoided are estimated or measured to be high (line A), the net cost savings from the intervention will be large (ΔA). Cost-benefit analysis of the inter-

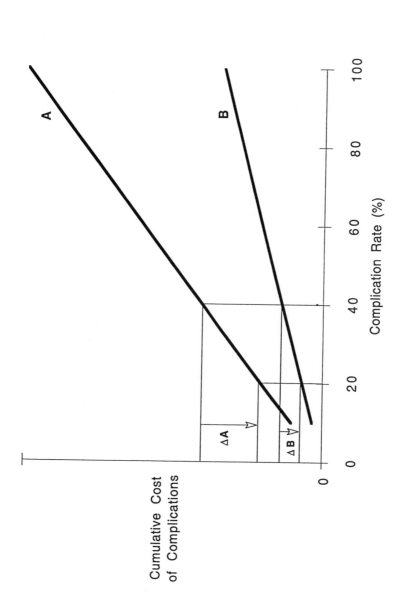

Figure 6-3 Sensitivity analysis. An example illustrating the sensitivity of the conclusions of a cost-benefit analysis to the value of one parameter (the estimated average cost of one complication).

vention will depend upon the accuracy of the measurement or estimate of the cost per complication; that is, the analysis is *sensitive* to the value of the cost per complication. Note that the absolute cost of complications in the example is sensitive to the complication rate. The higher the estimated or measured complication rate, the greater the absolute cumulative cost of complications. Outcomes studies that are robust (relatively insensitive to the exact value of important parameters) are generally more reliable, because even large differences between the measured (or estimated) and true value of the parameters have only small effects on the results of the analysis.

OUTCOMES METHODS IN CLINICAL PRACTICE

As noted previously, the factors motivating development of the outcomes movement include: concern that cost-containment efforts may adversely affect quality of care; need to specify to payers (especially insurance companies and managed care organizations) the quality of services being purchased; and the desire to reduce wasteful use of medical resources without limiting appropriate use of procedures and technologies. Outcomes research generally refers to large studies conducted to investigate global issues, but the topics of cost containment, marketing of services to managed care providers, and quality assurance are also important to individual practitioners and institutions. Furthermore, major revisions in the Joint Commission on Accreditation of Healthcare Organizations' *Comprehensive Accreditation Manual for Hospitals*, particularly with its sweeping changes in the way nutrition care of patients is evaluated, effectively require that individual institutions adopt an outcomes-oriented approach to continuing quality improvement.[41] Following is a presentation of some principles and examples of successful application of outcomes methods to clinical and institutional issues.

Principles

The principles discussed below can guide the successful application of outcomes research methods to clinical practice (see Exhibit 6–2). Underlying all of these principles is the admonition to *be practical*. Practitioners should initiate a project only if they have the experience, expertise, and

Exhibit 6–2 Principles for Applying Outcomes Research Methods to Clinical Practice

---

- Collaborate with acknowledged experts.
- Use established data collection resources.
- Use appropriate sampling techniques.
- Target tractable problems.
- Target big-payoff problems.
- Demonstrate effects of interventions with follow-up studies.
- Communicate results of outcomes studies and follow-up studies.
- Focus on outliers.

---

resources to complete the project successfully within a reasonable time frame.

Collaborate with Acknowledged Experts

Seek out people who are knowledgeable about the problem being studied. Taking advantage of other peoples' expertise with techniques such as study design, statistical analysis, database design and implementation, and clinical care saves time and improves the quality of outcomes projects.

Use Established Data Collection Resources

One of the most resource-intensive aspects of outcomes studies is collection of raw data. Use of available resources to facilitate data collection (including staff nurses, inpatient dietitians, utilization review staff, medical records, admissions office data files, physician consultants, and pharmacy records and personnel) is efficient and effective. It is easier to collaborate with someone who already has access to the needed data than to devote limited resources to collect data independently. Conversely, ease of availability of data should not dictate the outcomes that are analyzed. Measure what is important, developing cost-effective and time-effective data collection methods and resources when necessary.

Use Appropriate Sampling Techniques

Data collection can be prohibitive if information is sought on all patients. Choose appropriate samples (including proper mixes of medical and surgical patients, pediatric and adult patients, intensive care unit and floor care unit patients) to answer important questions without having to collect unmanageable amounts of information.

Target Tractable Problems

Do not identify problems that are beyond solution. For example, it is not helpful to document that lengths of stay are unnecessarily prolonged by the inefficiency of a home care company unless the means are available to change that company's practices or contract with a new vendor. Study outcomes and care processes that can be modified with certainty and cost-effectively.

Target Big-Payoff Problems

Study outcomes that, if improved, will have a major impact upon quality of care or costs. Changes that result in decreased lengths of stay are likely to have major financial consequences. Similarly, studies that demonstrate that simple changes in practice procedures can reduce cost without altering outcomes (eg, changing intravenous tubing every 48 hours rather than every 24 hours) have no downside and are often simple to implement.

Demonstrate Effects of Interventions with Follow-Up Studies

If an outcomes study leads to implementation of practice changes, restudy the outcomes after a suitable period of time to validate and conclusively demonstrate the benefits of the new practices.

Communicate the Results of Outcomes Studies and Follow-Up Studies

Improved quality of care and cost reduction are "marketable" to other clinicians, institutional administrators, and third-party payers. Demonstration of improved outcomes can be marketed to managed care providers to attract new contracts. Similarly, improved outcomes can be marketed to supervisors and administrators to justify the utility of specialized care activities and to garner additional resources to expand professional practice.

Focus on Outliers

Understanding a final conceptual issue can help practitioners select problems that are tractable, have a potentially big payoff, are easy to communicate and follow up, and are amenable to study using small samples of patients. In undertaking an outcomes study directed at producing a beneficial intervention, one can (1) target the entire population at risk for an adverse outcome and attempt to improve the average outcome across the whole population (improve the mean), or (2) study the subset of patients with adverse outcomes and attempt to reduce the number of especially poor outcomes (eliminate the outliers, see Figure 6–4). The first approach is appealing because it can improve the care of all patients. Its disadvantages are that data must be collected on all patients at risk (or a large, representative sample) and an intervention must be applied to the entire population. By focusing on the patients with the worst outcomes (outliers), the second approach significantly reduces the scope of an outcomes project and simplifies the design and implementation of the subsequent intervention. An additional advantage of the outlier approach relates to the payoff. It is generally true that patients with the worst outcomes also incur the highest cost. By targeting this subsegment of the entire at-risk population, the resulting intervention can be small in scope (directed at only a relatively small number of patients) and generate a disproportionately large payoff (because of the disproportionately high cost of the care of the outliers).

Examples

The principles articulated above are exemplified by the following three outcomes research projects. These three examples show how outcomes research can be applied to influence clinical practice and resource allocation in local settings. All three studies were conducted without financial support. They were all conceptually simple. They studied specific outcome parameters that had clinical, administrative, and financial relevance. None of the studies required more than 25 hours of staff time to complete. All of them led to improved patient care. They were also "marketed" to improve relationships with clinical services, to engender wider understanding of the role of a nutrition support service, and to solidify and increase financial and administrative support for clinician and team functions. One project was of sufficient scope and rigor to merit publication; the others were not of publication quality but were influential in the institution.

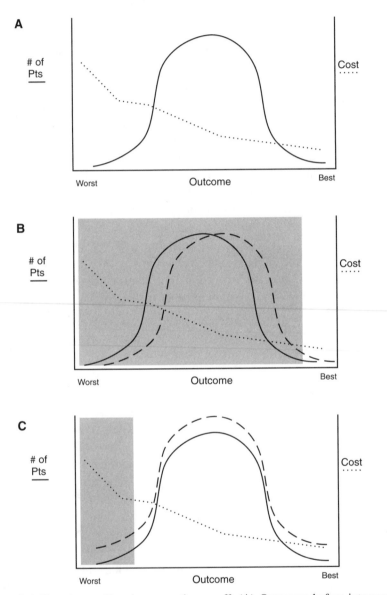

Figure 6–4 Targeting outliers increases the payoff. (**A**) Outcomes before intervention. (**B**) Outcomes following intervention when entire patient population is targeted. (**C**) Outcomes following intervention when outliers (patient with the worst outcomes) are targeted.

Home Parenteral Nutrition for Patients with Inoperable Malignant Bowel Obstruction

A hospital-based nutrition support team (NST) was concerned with the effort and resources required to administer home parenteral nutrition (HPN) to terminally ill cancer patients with inoperable malignant bowel obstruction (IMBO). Particularly problematic was the number of referrals from the gynecologic oncology service for HPN for patients with inoperable carcinomatosis from ovarian cancer. The team undertook a retrospective study to determine whether HPN for IMBO is beneficial (ie, Does it improve quality of life with a low complication rate?) and to determine the appropriate indications for HPN in these patients.[42] The team believed that quality of life was important, but its assessment was problematic. Many patients had already died, and the team felt it was too intrusive to contact families of former patients. To overcome these obstacles, the NST chose to review charts and NST records to reconstruct the team's perceptions and patient and family perceptions of the benefits of HPN in 17 patients. The team believed that for the purposes of the study, this methodology represented a good compromise between analytical rigor and the time and effort the team was able to commit. From the study, the team learned that most patients and families felt that HPN had been beneficial; the NST agreed with those perceptions in most cases (see Figure 6–5). In addition, the team learned that HPN for IMBO was most beneficial for patients with an expected survival of greater than 40 days and with strong family support who had failed aggressive pharmacologic interventions aimed at managing the symptoms of IMBO. Although this study was ultimately published, its real strength was its effect institutionally. As a result of the study, the institution allowed additional hours of pharmacist time to support this labor-intensive therapy. The study also provided data to present to the gynecologic oncology service to demonstrate why the NST was improving the quality of patient care by electing *not* to provide HPN to many ovarian cancer patients with IMBO; the data demonstrated convincingly that it was a futile undertaking in many patients.

The Impact of a Nutrition Support Team on Neonatal Nutrition Care

A hospital-based NST was concerned with the perception of its role in the institution's neonatal intensive care unit (NICU). Team members took advantage of an opportunity to perform a small outcomes study to demon-

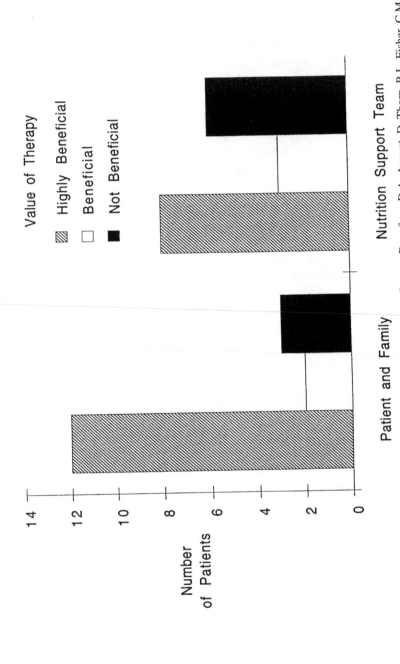

Figure 6–5 Perceptions of the value of home parenteral nutrition therapy. *Source:* Data from D.A. August, D. Thorn, R.L. Fisher, C.M. Welchek, Home Parenteral Nutrition for Patients with Inoperable Malignant Bowel Obstruction, *Journal of Parenteral and Enteral Nutrition,* Vol. 15, pp. 323–327, 1991.

strate the effectiveness of the NST in the NICU when temporary staff absences prevented the NST from completing regular rounds in the NICU for a 2-month period.[43] The team performed a retrospective review, comparing nutritional intake and length of total parenteral nutrition (TPN) therapy between a group of neonates ($N = 25$) treated with TPN after NST staffing was normalized (permitting participation in regular NICU rounds) and a group of neonates treated with TPN during the hiatus in rounds ($N = 28$). Information was abstracted from a review of charts and from data maintained in the pharmacy. Although little difference was observed in nutrient intake, the newborns who received TPN while the team participated in rounds had a significantly shorter duration of TPN therapy (see Table 6–4). These data provided convincing evidence to NICU practitioners of the utility of a NST participation in NICU rounds. The data were also used to support a NST request for supplemental staffing during temporary absences by demonstrating how the investment in personnel could pay for itself through reduced costs of nutrition support.

Improved Physician Compliance with Nutrition Team Recommendations

The parenteral and enteral nutrition team at the University of Michigan Hospitals developed a new TPN order form with the goals of reducing the use of expensive, nonstandard TPN formulations and increasing physicians' compliance with the team's TPN recommendations. The new order form made it more cumbersome for physicians to order nonstandard TPN formulas while making it easier to order two standard TPN formulas. The new order form also contained a box for team recommendations (recommendations were formerly written in progress notes); the recommenda-

---

Table 6–4 Impact of Parenteral and Enteral Nutrition (PEN) Team Rounds on Duration of Parenteral Nutrition Therapy in a Neonatal Intensive Care Unit

Neonates Requiring TPN (N)	Percentage of Patients off TPN by Day 22
No PEN team monitoring (28)	32
PEN team monitoring (25)	64

Source: Reprinted from T. Han-Markey, D.A. August, R. Schumacher. Impact of the nutrition support team (NST) on neonatal nutrition care. ASPEN 18th Clinical Congress, 1994 (Abstract).

tions were recorded by team clinicians before the physicians received the form to fill in new TPN orders. The last 100 patients for whom TPN was ordered using the old form were compared with the first 100 patients using the new form.[44] Use of the new form increased physicians' compliance with team recommendations by almost 50%. If increased compliance with expert recommendations is an appropriate intermediate end point for improved nutrition care, the data suggest that the new form facilitated improved patient care. Furthermore, with the new order form, use of non-standard TPN formulas decreased by one half (see Figure 6–6). The team projected that this change would save approximately 1000 hours of TPN compounding time yearly, with a resultant savings of approximately $20,000 annually. They concluded that simple clerical changes in the TPN order form resulted in both improved quality of care and reduced costs.

SUMMARY

Outcomes research is a powerful tool that is likely to play a major role in guiding health care reform. The methods of outcomes research are crucial weapons in the fight to prevent changes in the U.S. health care system from adversely affecting patient outcomes, the clinician-patient relationship, and the professional roles and activities of nutrition support practitioners. Nutrition support professionals must understand outcomes methodology and study interpretation if they are to prevent governmental agencies and third-party payers from misusing outcomes data to restrict reimbursement and from improperly disseminating misleading information concerning provider-specific quality and cost of care. Nutrition support professionals must also guard against the use of outcomes studies to formulate practice guidelines that limit freedom to make informed, individualized choices with and for patients. With an understanding of this global methodology and a commitment to adapt it to local practice settings, outcomes research can be applied to reduce costs and improve the quality of care.

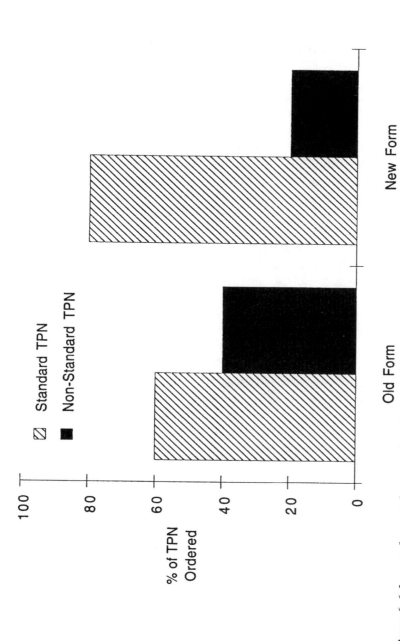

Figure 6–6 Impact of new total parenteral nutrition order form. *Source:* Data from A. Perez, C. Braunschweig, D. Kovacevich, and D.A. August, Improved MD Compliance with Nutrition Team Recommendations Using a Revised TPN Order Form, ASPEN 17th Clinical Congress, 1993 (Abstract).

REFERENCES

1. Epstein AM. The outcomes movement—Will it get us where we want to go? *N Engl J Med.* 1990;323:266–270.

2. Relman AS. Assessment and accountability: The third revolution in medical care. *N Engl J Med.* 1988;319:1220–1222.

3. Ellwood PM. Shattuck Lecture. Outcomes management: A technology of patient experience. *N Engl J Med.* 1988;318:1549–1556.

4. Tanenbaum SJ. What physicians know. *N Engl J Med.* 1993;329:1268–1270.

5. Sage WM. Outcomes research. *N Engl J Med.* 1994;330:434–435. Letter to the editor.

6. Bailit H, Federico J, McGivney W. Use of outcomes studies by a managed care organization: Valuing measured treatment effects. *Med Care.* 1995;33:AS216–AS225.

7. Wennberg J, Gittelsohn A. Small area variations in health care delivery. *Science.* 1973;182:1102–1108.

8. Wennberg JE, Freeman JL, Culp WJ. Are hospital services rationed in New Haven or over-utilised in Boston? *Lancet.* 1987;1:1185–1189.

9. Twomey PL, Patching SC. Cost-effectiveness of nutritional support. *J Parenteral and Enteral Nutr.* 1985;9:3–10.

10. Eisenberg JM, Glick H, Hillman AL, et al. Measuring the economic impact of perioperative total parenteral nutrition. *Am J Clin Nutr.* 1988;47:82–91.

11. ASPEN Board of Directors. Definition of terms used in ASPEN guidelines and standards. *J Parenteral and Enteral Nutr.* 1995;19:1–2.

12. King AB. Measurement of nutrition and health care outcome. *Nutr.* 1993;9:568.

13. Merkens BJ. Measuring outcomes of nutrition intervention. *J Can Diet Assoc.* 1994;55:64–68.

14. Cerra FB, McPherson JP, Konstantinides FN, Konstantinides NN, et al. Enteral nutrition does not prevent multiple organ failure syndrome (MOFS) after sepsis. *Surgery.* 1988;104:727–733.

15. Moore FA, Feliciano DV, Andrassy RJ, et al. Early enteral feeding, compared with parenteral, reduces postoperative septic complications. The results of a meta-analysis. *Ann Surg.* 1992;216:172–183.

16. American College of Physicians position paper. Parenteral nutrition in patients receiving cancer chemotherapy. *Ann Intern Med.* 1989;110:734–736.

17. Blaiss MS. Why outcomes? *Ann Allergy Asthma Immunol.* 1995;74:359–360.

18. Gabel J, Liston D, Jensen G, Marsteller J. The health insurance picture in 1993: Some rare good news. *Health Aff.* 1994;13:327–336.

19. Hannan EL, Kilburn H Jr, Racz M, et al. Improving the outcomes of coronary artery bypass surgery in New York State. *JAMA.* 1994;271:761–766.

20. Chassin MR, Hannan EL, DeBuono BA. Benefits and hazards of reporting medical outcomes publicly. *N Engl J Med.* 1996;334:394–398.

21. The Nordic Gastrointestinal Tumor Adjuvant Therapy Group. Expectancy or primary chemotherapy in patients with advanced asymptomatic colorectal cancer: A randomized trial. *J Clin Oncol.* 1992;10:904–911.

22. Coffey RJ, Richards JS, Remmert CS, et al. An introduction to critical paths. *Qual Manage in Health Care.* 1992;1:45–54.

23. Schriefer J. The synergy of pathways and algorithms: Two tools work better than one. *Joint Commission J on Qual Improvement.* 1994;20:485–499.

24. Dubois RW, Rogers WH, Moxley JH, et al. Hospital inpatient mortality: Is it a predictor of quality? *N Engl J Med.* 1987;317:1674–1680.

25. Greenfield S, Aronow HU, Elashoff RM, et al. Flaws in mortality data: The hazards of ignoring comorbid disease. *JAMA.* 1988;260:2253–2255.

26. Green J, Wintfeld N, Sharkey P, et al. The importance of severity of illness in assessing hospital mortality. *JAMA.* 1990;263:241–246.

27. Park RE, Brook RH, Kosecoff J, et al. Explaining variations in hospital death rates: Randomness, severity of illness, quality of care. *JAMA.* 1990;264:484–490.

28. Green J, Passman LJ, Wintfeld N. Analyzing hospital mortality: The consequences of diversity in patient mix. *JAMA.* 1991;265:1849–1853.

29. Blumberg MS. Risk adjusting health care outcomes: A methodologic review. *Med Care Rev.* 1986;43:351–393.

30. Green J, Passman LJ, Wintfeld N. Analyzing hospital mortality: The consequences of diversity in patient mix. *JAMA.* 1991;265:1849–1853.

31. Khuri SF, Daley J, Henderson W, et al. The National Veterans Administration surgical risk study: Risk adjustment for the comparative assessment of the quality of surgical care. *J Am Coll Surg.* 1995;180:519–531.

32. Roos LL, Sharp SM, Cohen MM, et al. Risk adjustment in claims-based research: The search for efficient approaches. *J Clin Epidemiol.* 1989;42:1193–1206.

33. Rontal R, Kiess MJ, DesHarnais S, et al. Applications for risk-adjusted outcomes measures. *Qual Assurance in Health Care.* 1991;3:283–292.

34. DesHarnais S, McMahon LF, Jr, Wrobleski R. Measuring outcomes of hospital care using multiple risk-adjusted indexes. *Health Serv Res.* 1991;26:425–445.

35. Concato J, Feinstein AR, Holford TR. The risk of determining risk with multivariable models. *Ann Intern Med.* 1993;118:201–210.

36. Jencks SF, Daley J, Draper D, et al. Interpreting hospital mortality data. The role of clinical risk adjustment. *JAMA.* 1988;260:3611–3616.

37. Charlson ME, Pompei P, Ales HL, et al. A new method of classifying prognostic comorbidity in longitudinal studies: Development and validation. *J Chronic Dis.* 1987;40:373–383.

38. Fetter RB, Youngsoo S, Freemen JL, et al. Case mix definition by diagnosis-related groups. *Med Care.* 1980;18(Feb suppl):1–39.

39. Marshall G, Grover FL, Henderson WG, et al. Assessment of predictive models for binary outcomes: An empirical approach using operative death from cardiac surgery. *Stat Med.* 1994;13:1501–1511.

40. Clintec Nutrition Company. *Cost Containment through Nutrition Intervention*. Deerfield, IL: Clintec Nutrition Company;1996.

41. Dougherty D, Bankhead R, Kushner R, et al. Nutrition care given new importance in JCAHO standards. *Nutr Clin Pract*. 1995;10:26–31.

42. August DA, Thorn D, Fisher RL, et al. Home parenteral nutrition for patients with inoperable malignant bowel obstruction. *J Parenteral and Enteral Nutr*. 1991;15:323–327.

43. Han-Markey T, August DA, Schumacher R. Impact of the nutrition support team (NST) on neonatal nutrition care. ASPEN 18th Clinical Congress; 1994. Abstract.

44. Perez A, Braunschweig C, Kovacevich D, et al. Improved MD compliance with nutrition team recommendations using a revised TPN order form. ASPEN 17th Clinical Congress; 1993. Abstract.

CHAPTER 7

Developing an Abstract
and Manuscript

Michele Morath Gottschlich

INTRODUCTION

Formal writing for professional audiences is a powerful communication tool. A myriad of opportunities exist for publishing nutrition-related information and research findings. The purpose of this chapter is to remove mental and emotional roadblocks from the minds of potential writers. This chapter reviews why, what, where, when, and how to produce a quality publication. It contains specific directions and tips for writing abstracts and manuscripts. Finally, it examines some strategies to guide the new author through the publication process.

WHY PUBLISH?

After completing a project or attending a conference, or perhaps after reading an article in a professional journal, many potential writers have thought, "I ought to write an abstract or article about . . . ." For many of us, that is as far as we go. Too many good research studies or clinical observations are never reported. That is unfortunate for several reasons. First, all of us have expertise that should be shared. Contributions to the body of existing scientific knowledge is vital for technical progress within the medical community.

Second, writing provides many personal benefits. The researcher or practitioner will likely benefit from producing an abstract or manuscript, because he or she will sharpen intellectual skills in the process. Furthermore, writing garners recognition from peers and fosters an increased awareness of talents by supervisors. Many organizations, particularly academic institutions, use publications and presentations as justification for professional advancement. Other institutions may approve travel funds to a meeting only if the employee is fortunate enough to have an abstract accepted. Perhaps the best reason to write, however, is having something worthwhile to say that may ultimately produce improvements in health care. Abstracts and manuscripts are excellent vehicles for disseminating information to colleagues. But, for any of these aforementioned benefits to be realized, individuals must share their work.

WRITING THE ABSTRACT

A good place to begin a discussion of writing is to consider the process of writing abstracts.[1–8] This information is useful for a number of reasons. Many of the guidelines for preparing abstracts can also be applied to manuscript writing, because the components of an abstract represent the backbone of a research paper. Abstracts often serve as the introduction to technical reports, manuscripts, and grant applications; as such, they may represent a significant factor in decisions to accept the work for presentation, publication, or funding. Familiarity with the components of an abstract can help readers—even those who are not interested in writing—quickly survey and/or critically evaluate the literature. Furthermore, abstracts are an important means of accessing articles in computerized document-retrieval systems. And finally, abstracts are often submitted to compete with many other abstracts for the honor of presenting a brief oral report[9] or poster[4,10] at a national meeting before the work has been published in a professional journal.

Abstracts can be very challenging to write, and they often require many revisions. They must be succinct yet include the necessary details. It is important to omit all jargon, cliches, and excess verbiage. Because an abstract is usually limited by space or the number of words allowed, it must be carefully crafted and every word must be scrutinized carefully for its clarity, logic, relevance, meaning, and impact.

COMPONENTS OF AN ABSTRACT

A scientific abstract has all the conventional components of a research manuscript; it simply condenses and summarizes the essential information and is usually written as one paragraph in the past tense. The format is fairly standard. It includes a title, introduction, purpose, study design, results, and a brief discussion of applications or conclusions.

The title is important because it is the most widely read part. The title should be short, specific, and informative. It should, in the fewest possible words, describe the content of the abstract. The title may not necessarily indicate what the abstract concludes, but it should at least convey what the abstract covers.

The introduction quickly gives an impression of the author's skill as an investigator and writer. The lead sentence should succinctly assert the overall purpose or rationale for the investigation. It should capture the reader's attention and interest by concisely highlighting the issue of concern. The introduction should end with the hypothesis. This section should provide a precise and specific description of the research question.

The introduction is followed by an account of the key elements of the study design and the technical methods used. This information should be brief yet sufficiently detailed so that the reader understands the experiment. The section describes the criteria for study enrollment, sample selection, and sample size; defines both the treated and control groups; and characterizes the experimental design (for example, the author would state here that the study was a prospective, randomized, double-blind clinical trial or a retrospective chart review). This section also indicates the procedures for data management. It is helpful to detail the statistical measures employed, such as t-tests, analysis of variance, stepwise regression, or chi-square analysis.

The most important part of the abstract is the results section.[6] This section is where the researcher summarizes the objective findings, which should either confirm or reject the hypothesis. When possible, numerical data with statistical analyses should be included. The author should provide exact values for more meaningful data (for example, mean +/− standard error). The word *significant* should be used only when documentation of statistical difference exists. The writer may elect to present information in tabular form if logic dictates and space permits.

The concluding sentence is the final component of the abstract. This statement answers the research question. It must relate to the study objectives and be supported by the results. One of the most common errors committed by new investigators is the failure to communicate their conclusions effectively. It is important to avoid overstatements and to avoid generalizing beyond the limits of the study design. For example, just because a particular intervention worked in the study sample does not mean that it will work in other patient populations. When drawing conclusions from research data, the investigator must recognize any limitations in the study design or its execution. If space permits, it may be appropriate to include new hypotheses derived from the data, but these should be very specifically identified as speculation. Some hint of future research may also be provided.

An abstract does not have room to include background information that led to the study, and it should not contain literature citations or footnotes. Abbreviations and acronyms can be used if they are defined or commonly used. However, the writer should avoid using them in the initial or concluding sentences; in the interest of time, many readers look at the first and last sentence and then decide whether to read the entire abstract. Thus, these two sentences must be completely clear.

REASONS ABSTRACTS ARE REJECTED

The abstract is scored by a committee of professionals who have significant expertise in the field. These individuals are usually very busy with many responsibilities and other distractions. They receive many abstracts to sort through, so an abstract should be of high quality. The author has only a few minutes to get a point across, so it is important to conform to all requirements. For example, one should never violate length restrictions. If guidelines require that the abstract be typed to fit a box of space on a special application form, then the author should stay within the designated line borders. This allows the abstract to be reproduced into proceedings or a publication. The author should avoid using product names if so requested. A smudged abstract filled with misspellings obviously works against the author. In many cases, poor presentation of information—not flawed research—is responsible for abstract rejection. Submissions can be disqualified for not following directions precisely or careless proofreading.[8] Common reasons for abstract rejection are listed in Exhibit 7–1.

Exhibit 7–1 Common Reasons Why Abstracts Are Rejected

- study methods not described
- inadequate sample size
- inadequate controls
- invalid statistics
- little or no objective data
- inaccurate data
- does not conform to typing format or rules specified by sponsoring organization
- poorly written, incoherent
- grammatical, syntax, or spelling errors
- nonstandard or undefined abbreviations
- identification of institution or authors in body of abstract
- conclusion not supported by the evidence
- no new information; findings of common knowledge
- data presented or published elsewhere
- insignificant study

ABSTRACT SCENARIO

Exhibit 7–2 represents a mock abstract that illustrates a number of common mistakes. Major concerns with this particular abstract include its lack of a purpose statement and its lack of substantive facts and data. Reviewers typically want to read details of the methods and results; for example, *diarrhea* and *delayed enteral support* should be defined, and statistics should be included to strengthen the abstract. Exhibit 7–3 illustrates a well-written mock abstract.[1,7]

WRITING THE MANUSCRIPT

If a research project is worth an abstract, it is probably ready to be developed into an article. However, research isn't all that is worthy of publication.[1,11] Potential writers should examine their own practice and realize that a diversity of publishing opportunities exist. Clinical observations, advancements in technology or care, case studies, teaching or cost-

Exhibit 7–2 Mock Abstract Likely To Be Rejected by Abstract Review Panel

SCIENTIFIC ABSTRACT REPRODUCTION FORM
(For *Original* Basic Research, Clinical and Outcomes Research)
Abstracts must be received by August 23, 1996

Important: Enclose original abstract plus 9 blinded copies. The blinded copies should contain only the abstract title and content, with authors' names and institution names under the abstract title deleted. No author names, institution names, or award selections should appear on the copies to ensure blind, objective review.

Contact Person - Type or print the following information *if author who should receive correspondence;* eliminate this information from blinded copies.

PLEASE PRINT

Name____Michele____M.____Gottschlich____PhD, RD, CNSD
   FIRST   INITIAL   LAST   DEGREE(S)

Mailing Address____Shriners Burns Institute____Nutrition
   INSTITUTION   DEPARTMENT

   3229 Burnet Avenue
   STREET ADDRESS

   Cincinnati____Ohio____45229–3095
   CITY   STATE   ZIP

Office Telephone (513) 872–6298   Home Telephone (513) 554–0100

FAX Number (513) 872–6999   Is the first author a member of A.S.P.E.N.? ☒ Yes ☐ No

EXAMPLE: (Do not use smaller type than in the example (typesize is 10 point)
THE ROLE OF ALUMINUM IN PARENTERAL NUTRITION-INDUCED BONE DISEASE. E.W. Lipkin, MD, PhD, S. Ott, MD, A. Chait, MD and D. Sherrard, MD, Department of Medicine, University of Washington, Seattle, WA
   Aluminum (Al) deposition in bone is associated with severe and disabling bone disease in the long-term parenteral nutrition (PN) patient.

Please consider my abstract for presentation in the following formats:
(see description of formats on other side)
☒ Paper presentation ☐ Poster presentation
   ☐ Either paper or poster
If my abstract is not accepted as either a paper or a poster, I would like it
to be considered for the Information Exchange. ☐ Yes ☐ No

Proof Your Abstract

Type abstract in box below being sure to STAY WITHIN BORDERS.
Please be sure to read the criteria on the reverse side and
the checklist at left prior to submitting your abstract

☒ *If Accepted for a paper presentation, I am a young investigator and wish to be considered for the Vars Research Award.*

☒ *If accepted, I wish to be considered for the Discipline Research Award. (A.S.P.E.N. members only)*
My discipline is: (Circle one)
Nurse · Dietitian · Pharmacist

ABSTRACT CHECKLIST:
Abstract will be used as camera copy. It must conform to the standards listed below or it will be rejected. Before mailing, check your abstract for the following:
☐ title is completely capitalized
☐ institutional affiliation and city are required
☐ no street address, zip, or grant support
☐ do not indent title
☐ stay within borders
☐ do not blacken borders
☐ justify left
☐ do not squeeze letters or lines
☐ no smudges or faint typing
☐ no underlining or capitalization for emphasis
☐ check for accurate spelling and hyphenation
☐ state conclusion; promise of additional data is unacceptable

DIARRHEA IN TUBE-FED BURN PATIENTS. M.M. Gottschlich, PhD, RD, M. Jenkins, RN, MBA, and G.D. Warden, MD Shriners Burns Institute, Cincinnati, OH
   The hypermetabolic state observed in thermally injured patients warrants aggressive nutritional management. Enteral support is the preferred route of nutrient delivery, however, diarrhea has been reported to be a major problem in hospitalized patients on tube feedings. The relationship of diarrhea to drugs, various tube feeding formulae (Osmolite HN, Traumacal, Ensure Plus, or a modular tube feeding), osmolality, specific nutrient intake, serum levels of vitamins and serum albumin was prospectively evaluated in 50 patients. The incidence of diarrhea was 32%. Drug therapy was a significant explanatory factor. Delayed enteral support was also associated with an increased incidence of diarrhea. Some tube feeding regimens were more frequently associated with absorption problems than others. Delayed enteral support was also associated with an increased incidence of diarrhea. Hypoalbuminemia, tube feeding osmolality, and serum vitamin A did not significantly correlate with diarrhea. We conclude that diarrhea is a major problem in patients on tube feeding.

Exhibit 7–3 Improved Version of Mock Abstract

Please read guidelines and instructions.
SCIENTIFIC ABSTRACT REPRODUCTION FORM
(For Basic and Clinical Research)
Abstracts must be received by August 28, 1992

Important: Enclose original abstract plus 9 copies. The copies should contain only the abstract box, with authors' names and institution names under the abstract title deleted. No author names, institution names, or award selections should appear on the copies to ensure blind, objective review.
Contact Person - Type or print the following information *of author who should receive correspondence*; eliminate this information from copies.

Name   Michele   M.   Gottschlich   PhD, RD, CNSD
    FIRST   INITIAL   LAST   DEGREE

Mailing Address   Shriners Burns Institute

    3229 Burnet Avenue

    Cincinnati   Ohio   45229-3095
    CITY   STATE   ZIP

Office Telephone(513) 872-6298   Home Telephone (513) 554-0100

FAX Number (513) 872-6999   Is the first author a member of A.S.P.E.N.? □ Yes   □ No

ABSTRACT RULES cont'd
12. Capitalize entire title. Do not underline author's names. Underlining or capitalization for emphasis in text is unacceptable. Single-space all typing (no space between title and body or between paragraphs). Indent each paragraph 3 spaces. Do not indent title. Brand names of products must not appear in titles.

13. Provide an original plus 9 copies. The copies should contain only the abstract box, with all award selections, contact person's name, author's names and institutions under the abstract title deleted. No author names, institution names, or award selections should appear on the copies to ensure blind, objective peer review.

14. No paper may be presented at the Clinical Congress if it has been published at any other national meeting prior to the date of presentation.

15. Submit abstract material and a check for $20.00 to A.S.P.E.N., 8630 Fenton St., Suite 412, Silver Spring, MD 20910. Fees must be submitted in U.S. dollars only; drawn on U.S. banks only.

EXAMPLE (Do not use type smaller than in example.)
THE ROLE OF ALUMINUM IN PARENTERAL NUTRITION-INDUCED BONE DISEASE. E.W. Lipkin, MD, PhD, S. Ott, MD, A. Chait, MD and D. Sherrard, MD Department of Medicine, University of Washington, Seattle, WA.
    Aluminum (Al) deposition in bone is associated with severe and disabling bone disease in the long-term parenteral nutrition (PN) patient.

PREFERENCE
✓ all that apply
☒ Scientific Short Paper Presentation only
□ Scientific Poster Presentation only
□ Either paper or poster
☒ If accepted, consider for Vars Research Award
☒ If accepted, consider for Discipline Research Award (A.S.P.E.N. members only)
✓ one: _____ Nurse
    _____ Dietitian
    _____ Pharmacist

ABSTRACT CHECKLIST
Abstract will be used as camera copy. It must conform to the standards listed below or it will be rejected. Before mailing, check your abstract for the following:
—title is completely capitalized
—institutional affiliation and city are required
—no street address, zip, or grant support
—do not indent title
—stay within borders
—do not blacken borders
—justify left
—do not squeeze letters or lines
—no smudges or faint typing
—no underlining or capitalization for emphasis
—check for accurate spelling and hyphenation
—state conclusion; promise of additional data is unacceptable

TYPE ABSTRACT IN BOX BELOW BEING SURE TO STAY WITHIN BORDERS

DIARRHEA IN TUBE-FED BURN PATIENTS. M.M. Gottschlich, PhD, RD, M. Jenkins, RN, MBA and G.D. Warden, MD Shriners Burns Institute, Cincinnati, OH
    The purpose of this prospective study was to determine factors associated with diarrhea (defined as >4 stools/day or a large, liquid stool >200 g) in tube-fed (TF) burn patients. Of the 50 patients studied, 16 (32%) developed diarrhea. Although the risk of diarrhea was associated with antibiotics ($p<0.05$), several nutrients also had an impact. Results demonstrated a significant relationship between dietary lipid ($p<0.05$) or vitamin A intake ($p<0.001$) and diarrhea. Implementation of TF within 48 hours post burn was also associated with decreased incidence of diarrhea ($p<0.001$). This presentation describes a modular TF program in which diarrheal frequency is lessened ($p<0.0001$). Hypoalbuminemia, TF osmolality, drugs used to prevent stress ulcers and serum vitamin A were irrelevant. The diarrheagenic nature of commercial TF appears to be the result of suboptimal diet therapy formulations. Further investigation will elucidate whether a) changes in prostaglandin generation/enhanced water and electrolyte losses related to ingestion of a high fat diet or b) histopathologic effects of retinoids or delayed feeding on intestinal mucosa are involved in the modulation of diarrhea. It is concluded that a low fat (<20% of kcal intake), vitamin A enriched (>10,000 IU/day), early enteral support program maximizes conditions which promote TF absorption during the nutritional rehabilitation of burns.

containment techniques, and new product trials all represent excellent materials for an article.

WHO SHOULD PUBLISH?

Who should publish a manuscript? Many health care professionals claim that they want to write, but they are intimidated by the process and the mystique associated with publishing. For some reason, publishing is often viewed as an unattainable goal, or something that others with more experience do. For many people, this apparent lack of confidence with regard to writing continues long after they are comfortable in their careers. Many potential authors have dismissed any notion of attempting to write for publication because they are convinced that they do not have the necessary time, background information, skills, or award-winning solutions. This attitude needs to change. One of the purposes of this chapter is to encourage readers to write and submit original papers of their own.

WHEN TO WRITE

One of the most frequent excuses offered by clinicians for not writing is "I can't fit it into my schedule." Some clinicians expect time to be allocated during their normal workday to write. Unfortunately, publishing is often not documented as a component of a health care job description. Some clinicians become experts at time management in an effort to devote a small portion of their workday to writing. But potential writers should realize that, initially, most of the time they invest will be their own time, away from the workplace. As a clinician develops a reputation as a writer, it may be possible to devote more approved work time to writing. However, widely published individuals typically are not 9-to-5 professionals. Their motivation is not their hourly wage, but the satisfaction derived from the process of sharing observations and findings.

WHAT TO PUBLISH

Writers should select a topic of keen interest to them, because they will be spending a lot of time analyzing the subject as they prepare a publication. It is important not to select a topic that is too broad, because this makes the writing process extremely difficult. Focus the topic.

Deciding what to publish requires familiarity with the literature. This is an important preliminary step because a journal's decision to accept a paper often hinges on whether the message is new in the literature. Even if the subject matter or findings are not new, the manuscript may get published if it expands on, disputes, or substantiates a previously published paper. Therefore, deciding what to write should depend in part on what one finds in the literature review.

HOW TO PUBLISH

There are two main facets to producing a manuscript for publication: (1) organizing thoughts logically and (2) expressing concepts clearly. A valuable prewriting technique that can help the writer achieve these desired outcomes is the preparation of an outline of the article. It establishes a sense of organization, defines the scope of the article, and helps the concepts flow in an orderly fashion. Yet the framework is flexible, so new thoughts can be easily incorporated before serious writing begins.

After the author has completed a simple outline of the major points, the next step is to develop each part. Beginning the document is the most difficult hurdle. Each author eventually figures out a preferred way to write. Some authors type first drafts themselves using a word-processing program. Others, especially born talkers, like to dictate for transcription by a typist. Others prefer paper and pen. The new author should select a writing medium that he or she feels comfortable with.

In the first draft, some authors elect to vigorously build a foundation with basic information and essential facts while ignoring grammar, spelling, punctuation, references, and editorial niceties. Others prefer to worry about details and perfect one paragraph of the paper at a time. It is up to the individual author to decide which method works best. The immediate goal, however, is to try to complete a first draft as quickly as possible; this provides a sense of the whole, from which the author can generate improvements.

The first draft should contain the major points, discussion, and conclusions. When the first draft is completed, the author should put it away for a week or so. Time gives perspective and makes it easier for a writer to be objective about what he or she has written. Defects, sloppy passages, and omissions become obvious, and often the writer has new ideas. The author should work on successive drafts and assess the paper for length, appropriateness of paragraph breaks, sentence clarity, adherence to the rules of syntax and grammar, logic in the sequence of ideas, adequate development of each major point, and good transition between different ideas. The title should succinctly reflect what the paper conveys. Now is the time to spellcheck the document, to insert subheadings to facilitate a desired shift of attention, and to design tables and figures to illustrate the major points and enhance essential content. Writers who plan to reproduce material previously published elsewhere should write for permission at this stage.

Pertinent and updated references should be included so that the reader may refer to original papers as desired for further elaboration of a point within the manuscript. Reference citations should be prepared in precisely the style specified by the publication. Failure to follow this dictum suggests a carelessness that will cause reviewers and editors to be suspicious of other aspects of the paper, including details of the study itself. There are differences of opinion regarding how many references are optimal, and this varies according to the journal. Certainly authors should emphasize the most recent literature and use primary references whenever possible.

After the paper has been modified to the author's satisfaction, the author should circulate the paper to as many people as possible. He or she should ask coauthors, peers, and experienced researchers to proofread. Seeking constructive criticism is a good way to improve the quality of one's work. It is better that a friend provides brutal input than a journal's reviewer. Successive revisions that integrate suggestions from colleagues as appropriate will further polish the paper. It is not uncommon for a manuscript to require a number of revisions before a powerful and effective final draft is produced.

It is a false assumption that the editor of a journal will take the time to revise a worthwhile paper for publication if it is poorly written. This rarely occurs. The editor may perform minor editorial changes, but poor writing is usually viewed as an indication of inferior work.[12] Therefore, beginners should look for a mentor or use the assistance of a support group as they develop their skills.

AUTHORSHIP AND ACKNOWLEDGMENTS

Determining who should be included as an author can be a sensitive issue. In some cases, the medical director or department head may insist on inclusion as an author, even if he or she has not directly participated in the project. Authorship is not justified in situations where an individual's participation is solely limited to collecting data, obtaining funding, obtaining consents, performing routine diagnostic and therapeutic efforts, performing secretarial duties, or reviewing and commenting on the paper. Technical assistance or contributions would be more appropriately recognized in an acknowledgment.

Authorship implies substantive intellectual and/or practical contribution to the publication and constitutes responsibility for the content. The first or primary author must be able to ensure the originality and integrity of the data and premise on which the report is based. Additionally, the first author should be instrumental in the writing process. Whereas the first author has made the major contribution and is responsible for the validity of the entire manuscript, secondary authorship also conveys significant participation in the study and shared responsibility for the document's content.

WHERE TO PUBLISH

Choosing the right journal is an important step in the publication process.[1,7,11] Therefore, it is necessary to be familiar with the different types of publications (see Table 7–1). The author should select a journal whose style, prestige, and audience will suit the material most effectively. As a general guideline, scientific research should be sent to peer-reviewed or refereed journals. A refereed journal uses two to three reviewers to evaluate the quality of a paper and shares the reviewers' comments with the author. Descriptive reports and anecdotal experiences may be sent to professional journals, magazines, or newsletters. Other factors to consider when picking a journal are circulation, audience, editorial approach, and reputation.

The author needs to consider proper format when preparing the final manuscript. Each publication has its own format, and journals differ greatly in their requirements. This vital information is typically printed as "Instructions" or "Guidelines to Authors." All journals publish their

Table 7–1 Types of Publications

Classification	Description	Examples
1. Scientific journal	Usually emphasizes original research. An article is typically published only after it has undergone the peer-review process and, in most cases, been modified in response to suggestions. Indexed in *Index Medicus*.	*Journal of American Dietetic Association* *Journal of Parenteral and Enteral Nutrition*
2. Professional	Often not peer-reviewed. Content is usually more practice-oriented.	*Nutrition in Clinical Practice* *Perspectives in Applied Nutrition*
3. Newsletter	Frequently managed by an institution or organization. Newsletters often accept contributions and represent a good place for the novice writer to develop skills and gain confidence.	*Support Line RD Dietetic Currents*
4. Magazine/ newspaper	Articles are often written by staff members, by professional writers, or by invitation. Many frequently include material written by health professionals.	*USA Today Glamour Parents*
5. Book	In most cases, an author is invited by the editor or publisher to contribute a chapter in accordance with the book's mission. For these efforts, the author generally receives a complimentary book and/or small honorarium.	*Nutrition Support Dietetics Core Curriculum* *Research: Successful Approaches* *Contemporary Nutrition Support Practice*

Source: M.M. Gottschlich, Effective Communication Techniques, *Support Line*, Vol. XVI, No. 2, p. 6, © 1994, Support Line.

---

manuscript requirements. Some publish their guidelines in every issue; others do this only once or twice a year. Typical instructions may include page limits, headings and subheadings, reference style, and the number of manuscript copies requested by the journal. Some require that an electronic copy accompany a hard copy of the manuscript. It is very important to follow the instructions precisely. Because of their limited staffing and the volume of submissions, many journal editors are quite rigid in their manuscript requirements and may refuse to circulate to reviewers those submissions that do not adhere to journal specifications.

SUBMITTING THE FINAL MANUSCRIPT

After completing the final document, the author is ready to send it for review. Most journal editors find it helpful for an author to prepare a cover letter to accompany the manuscript (see Exhibit 7–4). The purpose of the submission letter is to provide the editor with some vital information about the author and the paper. The letter should identify the paper by its full title. The author may wish to explain briefly the importance of the topic to the journal's readership. If timing of the publication is particularly important, the author should state the reasons. The cover letter should document the inclusion of any enclosures, such as artwork, copyright agreements, and permissions to reproduce. The cover letter should also indicate any conditions for publication of the paper. Finally, the letter of transmission should make clear who is the corresponding author, along with this person's address, professional affiliation, phone number, e-mail, and fax number. Particularly helpful are any forewarnings of upcoming address changes.

Once an author has submitted the manuscript, he or she must be patient. The process of manuscript review can take 2 to 3 months. If an author has not heard anything within that time, it is reasonable to submit a letter of inquiry regarding the status of the manuscript. It is considered unethical to publish a document that has been submitted or published elsewhere.[13] After an author sends a manuscript to one journal, it is proper etiquette to wait until the acceptance status is clarified before sending it to another journal.

REACTING TO THE EDITOR'S DECISION

What will the editor's response be? Few authors receive immediate and unconditional approval. Acceptances are usually provisional, with the final determination predicated on the author's revisions in accordance

Exhibit 7–4 A Typical, but Fictional, Submission Letter

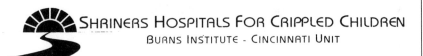

SHRINERS HOSPITALS FOR CRIPPLED CHILDREN
BURNS INSTITUTE - CINCINNATI UNIT

September 10, 1996

Elaine R. Monsen, PhD, RD
Editor, Journal of the American Dietetic Association
University of Washington, Mailstop DI-10
Seattle, Washington 98195

Dear Dr. Monsen:

Enclosed please find a full manuscript, diskette and four copies of
my work entitled **"Effect of Sleep on Energy Expenditure and
Physiologic Parameters in Critically Ill Pediatric Burn Patients."**
I have also included copies of permissions, copyright signatures
from all coauthors, and a 5 x 7 high resolution copy of each
illustration. My colleagues and I would like this manuscript
considered for publication in JADA as a research paper.

This is an investigation that really excites me. It is my vision
that the assessment and monitoring of sleep metabolism may
ultimately become a new horizon for dietitians -- yes, dietitians -
- because I hope that our work will eventually demonstrate that
sleep is nutrative and restorative, much in the same way as that of
essential nutrients! I hope you find this preliminary analysis to
be appropriate for the JADA readership.

Correspondence and phone calls about the paper should be directed
to me at the address and phone number below. My email address is
cinsbins@ix.netcom.com

Thank you for your consideration.

Sincerely,

Michele Gottschlich

Michele Gottschlich, PhD, RD, CNSD
Director, Nutrition Services

Courtesy of Shriners Hospitals for Children, Cincinnati, Ohio.

with the reviewers' criticisms. Not all suggestions for change must be accepted, but the author must be prepared to justify in a cover letter to the editor why he or she has not complied with the recommendations.

Rejection rates for prestigious journals are between 50% and 80%, so authors should not get angry or take disapproval personally. If comments accompany a rejection notice, the author should use them as a learning opportunity, heed the reviewers' advice when appropriate, and try again. It is worth noting that an excellent manuscript or abstract may be rejected simply because the timing was off. For example, an author who has had an abstract or manuscript rejected one year may resubmit the abstract unchanged the following year, and have it accepted. Perhaps the subject matter is not a good match for a particular journal at a particular time, or perhaps one of the reviewers has a personal bias against the theme. Another factor could be the backlog of manuscripts that a journal has already accepted for publication. Some articles are rejected by one journal only to be praised by another.

SUMMARY

Writing excellent abstracts or manuscripts is a skill that can be developed. It is not as difficult as it may seem. Careful consideration of the subject matter, as well as synthesizing information in an organized and clear manner is needed. Finally, a thorough understanding of publication guidelines and practices should allow clinicians to communicate effectively through these formats. The exuberance of completing a well-written document, seeing it in print, and realizing that one has made a contribution to the medical literature makes the effort worthwhile.

REFERENCES

1. Gottschlich MM. Effective communication techniques for the nutrition support dietitian: Developing the abstract, publication and presentation. *Support Line.* 1994;16:1–8.

2. Brown JM. Driven to abstraction: Writing an abstract for presentation or publication. *J Intraven Nurs.* 1989;12:326–328.

3. Ferrell BR. On writing abstracts. *Oncol Nurs Forum.* 1988;15:515–516.

4. Coulston AM, Stivers M. A poster worth a thousand words. How to design effective poster session displays. *J Am Diet Assoc.* Aug. 1993;93:865–866.

5. Baue AE. Writing a good abstract is not abstract writing. *Arch Surg.* 1979;114:11–12.

6. Warren R. The abstract. *Arch Surg.* 1976;111:635–636.

7. Zellmer WA. How to write a research report for publication. *Am J Hosp Phar.* 1981;38:545–550.

8. Rennie MJ. How to get your abstract accepted for ESPEN. *Clin Nutr.* 1994;13(suppl):62–64.

9. Garson A, Gutgesell HP, Pinsky WW, McNamara DG. The 10-minute talk: Organization, slides, writing and delivery. *Am Heart J.* 1986;111:193–203.

10. Thompkins DL. How to develop a poster. *J Intraven Nurs.* 1989;12:329–331.

11. Beare PG. Essentials of writing for publication. *J Opthalmic Nurs Tech.* 1988;7:56–58.

12. Kyllonen CF. Professional writing for medical professionals: Maintaining standards in technical communications. *Support Line.* 1994;16:9–10.

13. Puetz BE. 'Salami' publishing: When is enough enough? *Rehabil Nurs.* 1994;19:132.

CHAPTER 8

How To Prepare and Deliver Effective Oral Presentations

Michele Morath Gottschlich

INTRODUCTION

Oral presentation of results is an important component of the research process. One might think that verbal explanation would come naturally, in contrast to a more structured, written research report. But the fact is that both require hard work.[1] A formal lecture should be as well-planned and organized as a written document. Although much of the advice in Chapter 7 dealing with writing applies to planning an oral presentation, effective speakers need additional preparation in the areas of content and delivery. This chapter reviews the strategies for delivering presentations with confidence, credibility, and style.[1-8] It explains how to analyze the speaking situation. Then, it addresses key information regarding the preparation of the presentation. In addition, the chapter examines tips for relaxing physically and preparing mentally as well as methods for maximizing vocal and visual effectiveness. Finally, the chapter provides guidelines for handling questions and objections.

ANALYZE THE AUDIENCE AND SETTING

One of the first steps in preparing a presentation is to analyze the speaking situation.[1,6] The speaker can ask the person who invites him or her to characterize the audience and the event. Demographic information such as level of education or work experience, for example, will help the speaker ascertain the audience's needs. The speaker should establish whether there are any preliminary requirements such as preparing learning objectives, an outline, or a reference list for syllabus or continuing education applications.

Also, the speaker should try to obtain other key contextual variables in advance such as the anticipated number of participants, size of the room, the seating arrangement, and the timing of the presentation. This information helps to determine the formality and tone of the talk. In general, the larger the audience, the more formal the presentation. The larger the room, the more likely one would use a microphone and slides. If there are other speakers, the speaker should find out who else is speaking, the subject matter, and the order of the presentations. Then the speaker should prepare the talk accordingly.

ORGANIZE THE PRESENTATION

After analyzing the speaking situation, it is time to begin planning and organizing the content of the presentation using many of the guidelines for writing discussed in Chapter 7. The talk should be organized so that there is an opening, a body of major points, and a conclusion. A speaker should not feel compelled to tell the audience every little tidbit of information that he or she knows about a subject. Instead, the speaker should focus on a few main points and order them logically within the context of the lecture, taking into account the needs and expectations of the listeners. It is important to think about how to convey the information in a way that will interest the audience, to use explicit transitions, to summarize at the end of each point, and to introduce each new point clearly with statements such as "the second reason to support . . . ."

The speaker should give considerable thought to the introduction. It is an important time to establish competence, credibility, logic, and goodwill. Many speakers spend more time preparing and rehearsing their introduction than any other section of the speech. This is done for several reasons. First, the introduction is usually the best-remembered part of the presentation. Second, the opening shapes the listeners' expectations of what will follow. A speaker should let the audience know what will be covered during the allotted time; the audience should not have to guess what the main elements of the talk will be.

If possible, one should open with something interesting. Speakers use different approaches to capture the attention of their listeners. Some open with a pertinent quotation, controversial statement, compelling statistic, or rhetorical question. Others use humor or a personal anecdote related to the subject. Still others prefer to get right to work, addressing the audience without any dramatic or unusual introduction at all. There is no wrong or right way; each speaker should decide what will work best.

The conclusion is usually the second most-remembered part of a presentation. Here speakers can summarize the key elements of the message that they want listeners to understand or accept. Therefore, extra time and attention should be directed to its preparation.

When concluding a speech, it is usually appropriate to summarize briefly the key points of the presentation and tie them together. The conclusion should be the climax of the talk, but it should be succinct. Speakers who drag out a speech for more than several minutes after they have stated "in conclusion . . ." may seriously compromise all the good they have accomplished up to that point.

HOW TO REDUCE ANXIETY

Many people tremble at the thought of speaking in public. Being in front of a large crowd of people can be very anxiety-producing, primarily because of the tension or embarrassment associated with doing poorly while at the center of attention. One should not dwell on or magnify stage fright, or it can be debilitating. The anxiety can be controlled or minimized. Speakers should realize that a certain amount of nervousness is natural and can be facilitative. The excitement can be channeled to help the speaker express the ideas more energetically.

Fear usually peaks offstage. The empty minutes of anticipation prior to the presentation are the worst. Fortunately, there are ways to reduce jitters, or at least prevent the listeners from realizing that the speaker is tense.

- Try to concentrate on relaxing.
- Take a deep breath and hold it for 20 seconds, then release the breath slowly.
- Arch the back, stretch the arms, or clench the fists.
- Take a sip of water.
- Maintain a positive outlook.

In other words, one should view the situation as an opportunity for growth rather than a catastrophic event.

Another way to reduce anxiety is to be prepared. It is perfectly acceptable for speakers to use notes to help them remember items they wish to convey. Putting the information on paper eliminates some degree of nervousness, but the speaker should be familiar enough with the content that the talk is not read verbatim from notes. Some degree of spontaneity is more engaging for the audience and demonstrates a speaker's confidence. The speaker should practice the talk aloud so that the material becomes familiar. The more familiar a speaker is with the talk, the more confidence and poise he or she will exude. Practice also makes a speaker aware of the length of the speech and provides the opportunity to modify it so that it is within the established time frame. A good speaker never exceeds the time allotment.

The speaker should concentrate on talking at a rate that listeners can easily understand, and the speaker should appear relaxed. Pace the presentation so that it is not too fast or too slow. A fast pace can suggest that the speaker is not sensitive to the audience's needs. Conversely, a pace that is too slow may connotate a lack of mental acuity on the speaker's part. Some speakers tape record a practice session and count how many words they speak per minute. In general, a rate of 125 to 250 words per minute is easily understandable. Rehearsing also helps improve the speaker's fluency, exposes gaps in reasoning, and helps the speaker become more comfortable with the coordination of visual aids. The speaker's goal should be to know the talk well enough to be able to use a pointer to direct attention as appropriate to the visual aids.

Common sense will dictate how many times one needs to rehearse. Some speakers practice with their more supportive but toughest colleagues. Speakers who do this should listen to their colleagues' comments, try not to become discouraged or defensive, and make changes as appropriate.

When it is the actual day of the talk, the speaker can do a number of little things to reduce stress. Arrive at the room ahead of time to check it out. Observe the size of the room and the seating arrangements. Find out if the screen is to the left or the right. Determine how to get to the podium (some stages can only be entered by stairs from the left or right). Check the lectern to determine if there is sufficient light for scanning notes. See if the microphone is operational (tap it). Become familiar with the pointer.

Find the slide-advance button or the overhead projector on/off switch. If time permits, run through the slides quickly to be sure that they are positioned properly, although this should have been done previously in the speaker's "get ready" room.

SPEAKING ETIQUETTE

Arrive at the session early (the only thing worse than arriving late is not arriving at all). Introduce oneself to the moderator or host. Then be seated on the aisle near the front of the room. When the time comes to speak, walk confidently to the podium. After reaching the podium, smile and establish eye contact with the audience, scanning them from right to left. Allow the listeners a moment to focus their attention. Now address the moderators. Usually one of the moderators introduces the speaker. If Dr. A makes the introduction, say, "Thank you Dr. A; Dr. B, ladies and gentlemen . . . ." Then, acknowledge the occasion and express appreciation to the sponsor before launching into the talk.

VISUAL AIDS

Visual aids are an important accompaniment to oral presentations.[3,5,7] They help keep the talk interesting by providing a visual complement, they increase the amount of information retained by the listener, and they enhance the perception that the presenter is professional and credible. Create simple, neat, organized, and professional-looking visuals. Use phrases or short sentences to reinforce or outline main points. And make certain that visual aids pertain directly to the presentation.

The most frequently used visual aids in addressing audiences less than 50 people are chalkboards, flip charts or posters, transparencies displayed by an overhead projector, printed material (handouts), videotape or film, and physical props. Factors influencing the selection of teaching aids include the purpose of the presentation, audience size, location, budget, preparation time available, ability to reuse the visual aid in future presentations, and complexity of the message[7] (see Exhibit 8–1).

Researchers commonly use slides as a visual aid. Slides can be a very effective complement to the spoken word for larger audiences or scientific sessions. However, several basic rules must be observed.[5] Spellcheck all

Exhibit 8–1 Factors Influencing the Selection of Visual Aids

HANDOUTS

Advantages

- easy and quick to prepare
- inexpensive
- relieve audience from taking notes

Tip

- Establish who will photocopy and distribute.

FLIP CHARTS

Advantages

- easy and quick to prepare
- effective for small or informal audiences
- inexpensive
- can be easily adapted to change

Tip

- Establish who will supply paper and markers.

OVERHEAD TRANSPARENCIES

Advantages

- easy to prepare
- inexpensive
- easy to carry and store
- can be resequenced during presentation or written upon

Tips

- Establish who will supply projector.
- Ensure that a replacement bulb is available.

---

continues

Exhibit 8–1 continued

SLIDES

Advantages

- effective for large audiences
- routinely used for scientific sessions

Tips

- Establish who will provide projector.
- Determine who will provide slide carousel.
- Ensure that a replacement bulb is available.

---

slides; there is no excuse for typos. Do not overload slides with unnecessary details or excessive verbiage. Everyone in the audience should be able to read the slides. Many tables and figures appropriate for publication are too dense for slide presentation. It is inexcusable to say: "I know you probably can't read this slide because . . . ." If people in the audience will not be able to see the slide from the back of the room, do not use the slide.

The use of color can be an effective way of highlighting important points or accenting different sets of data. One certainly needs to consider color selection carefully when preparing visually appealing slides. On a dark background, light colors should be used; dark colors on a dark background (blue on black, for example) are difficult to discern. Although no specific colors are mandatory, several concepts should be kept in mind. Avoid using red and green whenever possible, because 5% of people are red/green color blind. In addition, one should avoid using too many colors, because this is confusing.

A frequent mistake is to include information on the slide that is not discussed in the presentation. Another common fault with the use of slide media is to read them verbatim. Slides should be used to extend the verbal presentation, not reproduce it. The usual time allotted is approximately 1 to 2 minutes per slide. Speakers who display someone else's data on a slide should put the name of the first author, journal, and year at the bottom of the slide. In addition, explanatory titles should accompany data slides to help orient the viewer to the general message. Other guidelines for the preparation of slides are reviewed in Exhibit 8–2.

It is wise to screen visual aids before the presentation to check for accuracy and readability. There is no excuse for presenting media out of sequence, upside down, or backwards. During the presentation, the speaker should always look at each transparency or slide to be sure it is the correct one. A good speaker must be comfortable with the possibility that it may be necessary to proceed with the presentation without the visual aids that are planned. The slide projector may jam, the overhead projector may blow a light bulb, or there may not be any chalk for the

---

Exhibit 8–2 Guidelines for Preparing Slides

- A horizontal format, using a ratio of 2 units of height for 3 units of width (ie, 6cm × 9cm), makes the best slides.
- Capital letters in a bold, simple typeface are easiest to read.
- Illustrations, graphs, and figures should be drawn in India ink on a white background.
- Use a simple design: do not put too much information on one slide.
- Do not exceed 50 spaces (including letters, spaces, and punctuation) per horizontal line.
- Do not exceed 7–10 lines of lettering or numbers per slide.
- Use maximum contrast between lettering and background: black on white, black on light yellow, white on blue.
- Limit each slide to one idea, even if it takes several slides to make your point.
- Allow an adequate margin on all sides.
- Legends on graphs, tables, and figures should be clear and legible.
- Color can be used to highlight points or accent different data sets.
- Complicated data can be supported with handouts.
- Proofread all material to avoid misspellings, which are distracting.
- Place a red dot or number on the lower left-hand corner of the slide when you hold it so that you can read it in proper position.
- Important features on an X-ray or photomicrograph should be pointed out with arrows or other symbols.
- Illustrations and photographs should be easily recognizable.

Source: © 1991, The American Dietetic Association. "Research: Successful Approaches." Used by permission.

blackboard. Be prepared to adjust to these contingencies in an easygoing fashion.

EFFECTIVE ORATION TECHNIQUES

Other suggestions for delivery include displaying a high level of expression and enthusiasm for the topic. A good speaker has life and color in his or her voice. Oral presentations are generally more interesting if the speaker conveys a conversational yet authoritative tone. Avoid the use of the verbal fillers "um," "uh," "you know," "like," "okay," and other such speech tics. These image killers make a speaker appear indecisive and lacking in knowledge and confidence.

Do not mumble. Enunciate. One's body language and tone of voice should match the message. Use gestures to reinforce points—such as raising one, two, or three fingers when counting ideas. Repeat key points, expand on complex issues, and be oneself. This is crucial to good public speaking. A person who never tells stories or jokes off the platform should not try it at the lectern. It will not be natural and, consequently, can backfire. If the presenter speaks and behaves naturally, audiences will be tolerant and supportive. Then, even if the presenter happens to tip over a glass of water, cough, or get cotton mouth, the audience will continue to appreciate the information the speaker is sharing.

During the presentation, be sure to look at the audience. Make an attempt to scan the entire room periodically. Maintaining good eye contact conveys sincerity and confidence. It also provides clues about whether the audience is understanding the message. And smile! It is important for the audience to think that the speaker is enjoying this!

RESPONDING TO QUESTIONS EFFECTIVELY

A question-and-answer period may follow the presentation. Many speakers experience anxiety over this type of exchange, perhaps because they have no knowledge or control over what the questions will be. Even after some practice with this type of dialogue, it may be intimidating to see a senior member of a society approach the microphone to ask a question or challenge one's beliefs. Relax. Try to learn something. Listen to the question carefully while establishing eye contact with the questioner.

Some people find it helpful to repeat the question to be sure they understand it precisely. This gives them some time to compose a response. Always repeat the question if the person asking it does not have a microphone, so that the entire audience can hear.

Then, keep the answers brief. It is much easier to get into trouble by saying too much than by saying too little. Remember that not everyone in the audience will share the questioner's interest in a particular aspect of the subject. Furthermore, a number of people may be waiting to ask questions. And one last reason for keeping the answers short is that they are easier for the audience to understand than long, rambling responses. Do not argue. Be direct, helpful, professional, and diplomatic when responding. Do not be afraid to express personal feelings in the comments. In most cases, the questioners are looking for the speaker's opinion rather than factual information. Almost invariably, a question will come up that the speaker is not prepared to answer. When a speaker does not know the answer, he or she should admit this; it is much better to acknowledge this predicament in a straightforward manner. One can ask for a business card and offer to get back with an answer if possible. Avoid bumbling your way through a response and pretending to be knowledgeable. And feel free to ask the audience to describe their experiences. If someone makes a very good point, be appreciative; however, it is unnecessary to say "thank you for that interesting comment" to everyone. Finally, it is polite to look at the audience when they applaud.

SUMMARY

Communicating the results of a research project is a critical step of the research process because it promotes knowledge and contributes to the improvement of practice. The ability to verbalize research findings effectively also helps to generate interest and resources for future studies and collaboration. Therefore, aversion to public speaking needs to be overcome if one is striving to be perceived as a leader in a given field.

Fortunately, good delivery style is a learned skill that can be developed over time with practice and experience. The strategies discussed above will help researchers to use the power of oral presentations to communicate knowledge and market research in an effective and interesting way. Researchers who are in the early stages of their careers should try to accept all invitations to speak, regardless of the size and prestige of the meeting. Accepting speaking engagements frequently leads to other invitations. And every new experience instills added confidence. Furthermore, speaking engagements allow researchers to improve their understanding of the subject and help them polish their delivery style while benefiting others with the knowledge they are sharing. Finally, don't expect perfection or too much enjoyment the first time. Both will come with practice. New speakers should view themselves as evolving human beings and realize that everybody makes mistakes. Just correct any errors immediately, if possible, and resolve to improve on that score the next time.

REFERENCES

1. Hawkins C. Oral presentation of results. *Br Med Oral Maxillofacial Surg.* 1984;22:365–367.

2. Matarese LE. The fine points of public speaking. *Support Line.* 1994;16:13–15.

3. Chernoff R. Techniques and approaches for presenting research data. In: Monsen ER, ed. *Research—Successful Approaches.* Chicago: The American Dietetic Association; 1992;375–388.

4. Clark TD. *Power Communication.* Cincinnati, OH: South-Western Publishing Co, 1994;1–339.

5. Hammerschmidt DE. Don't crowd your slides. *JAMA.* 1984;252:775–776.

6. Gottschlich MM. Effective communication techniques for the nutrition support dietitian: Developing the abstract, publication and presentation. *Support Line.* 1994;16:1–8.

7. Spinler SA. How to prepare and deliver pharmacy presentations. *Am J Hosp Pharm.* 1991;48:1730–1738.

8. Goodman N. The presentation of research in clinical practice. *Brit J Clin Pract.* 1990;44:345–347.

CHAPTER 9

Professional Obligations

Jon T. Albrecht

INTRODUCTION

Traditionally, professionals have not been required to follow stringent research guidelines when performing investigations involving foods and nutrition products. However, the advent of "pharmaconutrition," the use of nutrition products to achieve a pharmacologic effect, has caused this to change. In general, any product researched for its pharmacologic effect must comply with Food and Drug Administration (FDA) regulations. Pharmacologic effect is broadly defined as any chemical that affects living processes. Pharmaconutrition investigators must be aware of their responsibilities to substantiate their findings clearly.

Responsibility of the investigator goes well beyond the development of a research protocol. Responsibilities include the following:

- maintaining scientific objectivity
- collecting and recording data thoroughly
- submitting protocols that involve patients to institutional review board (IRB)
- protecting subjects from harm
- obtaining informed consent for every patient
- managing research funding with integrity
- presenting and publishing research in peer-reviewed media

PATIENTS' RIGHTS

The development of statements regarding patients' rights began after World War II as a result of the Nuremberg War Crimes Trials. The Nuremberg Code, published in 1947, addressed patient safety and investigator ethics in the context of research performed on concentration camp prisoners.[1] In 1994, the American Medical Association's Council on Ethical and Judicial Affairs defined the following fundamental patients' rights:

1. The patient has the right to receive information from physicians and to discuss the benefits, risks and costs of appropriate treatment alternatives. Patients should receive guidance from their physicians as to the optimal course of action. Patients also are entitled to obtain copies or summaries of the medical records, to have their questions answered, to be advised of potential conflicts of interest that their physicians might have and to receive independent professional opinions.
2. The patient has the right to make decisions regarding the health care that is recommended by his or her physician. Accordingly, patients may accept or refuse any recommended medical treatment.
3. The patient has the right to courtesy, respect, dignity, responsiveness and timely attention to his or her needs.
4. The patient has the right to confidentiality. The physician should not reveal confidential communications or information without the consent of the patient, unless provided for by law or by the need to protect the welfare of the individual or the public interest.
5. The patient has the right to continuity of health care. The physician has an obligation to cooperate in the coordination of medically indicated care with other health care providers treating the patient. The physician may not discontinue treatment of the patient as long as further treatment is medically indicated, without giving the patient sufficient opportunity to make alternative arrangements for care.
6. The patient has the basic right to have available adequate health care. Physicians, along with the rest of society, should

continue to work toward this goal. Fulfillment of this right is dependent on society providing resources so that no patient is deprived of necessary care because of an inability to pay. Physicians should continue their traditional assumption of a part of the responsibility for the medical care of those who cannot afford essential health care.[2]

INFORMED CONSENT

In accordance with recognized patients' rights, informed consent must be obtained before any subject may participate in a clinical investigation. The FDA, which has regulations governing informed consent, defines informed consent as "more than a signature on a form, it is a process of information exchange that includes recruitment materials, written materials, verbal instructions, question/answer sessions and measures of subject understanding."[3]

Informed consent should be obtained from subjects or their representatives who are competent to consider whether to participate or not participate in an investigation. The investigator should be careful to avoid coercion or undue influence in obtaining informed consent. Informed consent may not waive patients' rights. Written materials and verbal discussions should be appropriate for the subjects' level of understanding. If informed consent is to be obtained from non–English-speaking subjects, the written informed consent must be accurately translated to the appropriate language. Investigations that provide subjects with material compensation may not use completion of the investigation as a condition to receive full compensation. Compensation should be provided throughout the study; however, a portion may be reserved for payment upon completion. Consent forms may not imply that the investigation has been reviewed or approved by the FDA.

Elements of informed consent include the following:

1. A statement that the study involves research, an explanation of the purposes of the research, the expected duration of a subject's participation, description of procedures to be followed, and identification of any procedures which are investigational.

2. A description of any reasonable foreseeable risks or discomforts to the subject.
3. A description of any benefits to the subject or to others which may reasonably be expected from the research.
4. A disclosure of appropriate alternative procedures or course of treatment, if any, that might be advantageous to the subject.
5. A statement describing the extent, if any, to which confidentiality of records identifying the subject will be maintained and that notes the possibility that the Food and Drug Administration may inspect the records.
6. For research involving more than minimal risk, an explanation as to whether any compensation and an explanation as to whether any medical treatments are available if injury occurs and, if so, what they consist of, or where further information may be obtained.
7. An explanation of whom to contact for answers to pertinent questions about the research and research subjects' rights, and whom to contact in the event of a research-related injury to the subject.
8. A statement that participation is voluntary, that refusal to participate will involve no penalty or loss of benefits to which the subject is otherwise entitled, and that the subject may discontinue participation at any time without penalty or loss of benefits to which the subject is otherwise entitled.
9. Additional elements of the informed consent where appropriate:
   a. A statement that the particular treatment or procedure may involve risks to the subject (or to the embryo or fetus, if the subject is or may become pregnant) which are currently unforeseeable.
   b. Anticipated circumstances under which the subject's participation may be terminated by the investigator without regard to the subject's consent.
   c. Any additional costs to the subject that may result from participation in the research.
   d. The consequences of a subject's decision to withdraw from the research and procedures for the orderly termination of participation by the subject.

e. A statement that significant new findings developed during the course of the research which may relate to the subject's willingness to continue participation will be provided to the subject.

f. The approximate number of subjects involved in the study.[4, 5]

The common problems the FDA has found with informed consent documents include:[6]

- failure to include all the required elements specified in 21 CFR 50.25
- failure to explain technical/scientific language
- failure to state that the drug, biologic, or device is experimental
- failure to state *all* the purposes of the research
- failure to state the expected duration of the subject's participation
- overstated facts or overly optimistic tone or wording
- failure to describe completely the procedures to be followed
- failure to describe adequately the treatment alternatives available to the subject or the risks or benefits of the alternatives
- failure to describe accurately the extent to which confidentiality will be maintained, or failure to advise the subject that the FDA may inspect the records
- failure to describe the manner of payment, if any, to subjects
- failure to provide a contact for answers to questions about the research, research subjects' rights, and research-related injury to the subject (The contact names, telephone numbers, and addresses [when appropriate] should be included.)
- failure to include "additional elements of informed consent" when those elements are appropriate, or including certain elements when they are inappropriate
- omission of a written summary of what is to be said to the subject for IRB review when "short-form" written-consent documents are to be presented orally to subjects, or failure to provide the written summary to research subjects
- lack of study-specific information (use of "boiler-plate" forms)
- failure to obtain IRB review and approval prior to use

INSTITUTIONAL REVIEW BOARDS

It is the responsibility of the IRB to review and approve all clinical investigations. The IRB's primary purpose is to protect the rights and welfare of the subjects of clinical investigations. The IRB is charged to review and approve the research protocol. The research protocol includes the informed consent. The IRB must also review investigations in progress and ensure that no unauthorized changes have been made to the approved protocol.

The IRB consists of at least five members. The members of the IRB reflect a cross-section of the general population with varying backgrounds, professions, and sex. The members should be sensitive to cultural differences. The membership must include at least one nonscientist, at least one individual not related to the institution, and one layperson. The layperson must be present for all votes. Individuals involved in the clinical investigation may not vote. The institution may override the IRB's approval but may not override the IRB's disapproval.[5,7]

IRBs have written guidelines and procedures for the submission of clinical investigations for subsequent review and approval. Many IRBs provide questionnaires to aid the investigator in preparing protocols. Cornell University has published its guidelines on an Internet web site (http://www.osp.cornell.edu/UCHS-Guidelines.html). The investigator must answer the following questions:

- What is the pool of subjects?
- How are the subjects to be recruited?
- What is the risk to the subjects? Could the research be done without using humans?
- How will the subjects be informed that they do not have to participate in the study and that they may withdraw at any time with no penalty?
- In what ways have the confidentiality and privacy of the subjects' responses been ensured?
- Is there deception to the human subjects? If yes, what debriefing procedures have been arranged?
- What provisions have been made for cultural and language problems, if they arise?

The FDA monitors IRBs through the Bioresearch Monitoring Program. The Bioresearch Monitoring Program reviews an IRB's compliance with its own written policies and procedures, as well as with FDA guidelines.

CARE OF HUMAN AND ANIMAL SUBJECTS

An additional responsibility of the IRB relates to the care of human and animal subjects. Although review of the research protocol and the informed consent plays a large role in minimizing the risks to human and animal subjects, there are additional considerations.

The Public Health Service defines a human subject as "a living individual about whom an investigator (whether professional or student) conducting research obtains data through intervention or interaction with the individual or identifiable private information."[5] The definition of research involving human subjects also includes organs, tissues, and body fluids that are individually identifiable. Written, recorded, or graphic information that is individually identifiable is also included in the definition.

In its *Guide for the Care and Use of Laboratory Animals*, the Public Health Service outlines the necessary requirements for institutional policies, animal housing and care, veterinary care, and physical plant.[8] The IRB is responsible for ensuring that investigators adhere to these standards.

The investigator is required to report all adverse events occurring during the clinical investigation. The events are reported to the IRB and the study sponsor. Determination is then made regarding the significance of the adverse event and the need to discontinue or modify the study.

RECORDKEEPING

One of the most laborious responsibilities of the clinical investigator is recordkeeping. The investigator must maintain accountability records for drugs, biologics, and devices used in the research protocol. The records must include when the study materials were received from the sponsor and the disposition of all test materials (including wastage). The burden of proof is placed upon the investigator to provide all documentation necessary to demonstrate what materials were used on what subjects and that there was no diversion of study materials. Upon completion of the investigation, the investigator is responsible for returning any unused study materials to the sponsor. This establishes that subjects received the intervention outlined in the study protocol.

The investigator must keep records of the clinical investigation. The records are comprised of study protocol and related documentation and case history records. These records must be maintained for a period of time defined by the IRB and/or the FDA. The study protocol and related documentation records must contain the following elements:[9, 10]

- a statement of the study's objectives and purpose
- for studies of drugs (including biologics, medical foods, and food additives), each investigator's name, address, and statement of the qualifications, as well as each subinvestigator's name; the research facility's name and address; each reviewing IRB's name and address
- subject selection and inclusion criteria
- description of the study design, controls to be used, and procedures to minimize investigator bias
- drug dosage calculation, including the maximum dose and length of therapy
- description of observations and measurements to be made
- measures, including procedures of laboratory tests, used to minimize risks and monitor outcomes

The case history must contain the following elements:

- subject identification
- information that the subject meets selection criteria
- information on length of exposure to the study material(s)
- case report form submitted to the sponsor
- data to support information supplied on the case report form
- information from all tests and procedures; progress notes; consultation notes; correspondence; data on the subjects' clinical condition before, during, and after the clinical investigation; diagnoses made; and factors that might later affect the study materials

DATA COLLECTION TOOLS

Forms for data collection may be generated from a word processor and then photocopied or typeset for mass production. However, this practice makes it difficult to use the data after they have been collected. Many studies never see completion because the data are not in a readily usable, retrievable format. It is recommended that the investigator develop a plan before collecting data, to get the data into a database to facilitate retrieval and analysis. There are many alternatives to automate data collection and retrieval.

One method for automating data collection is to equip research personnel with palmtop or laptop computers. With database software installed, data can be collected and entered directly. A properly developed data application will facilitate consistency and continuity in data collection. Once collected, the data can be compiled, sorted, rearranged, and reported in a variety of different ways. Common brand names for database software include Access®, FoxPro®, and Paradox®. The advantages of this method of data collection are obvious. Data are collected and immediately available. The disadvantages are that, for a large study, equipping multiple researchers can result in large capital expenditures; one must consider the methods for merging data from multiple computers; and the researcher must develop a plan for data backup in the event of equipment failure.

Another method for automating data collection is to equip research personnel with barcode or lightpen equipment. Barcode and lightpen equipment allow personnel to collect data by answering multiple-choice questions. The advantages include uniformity in data collection and enhanced mobility due to the lightweight, portable nature of the equipment. Disadvantages include limited data collection capabilities, equipment durability, and large capital expense.

The most economical and flexible alternative for data collection is to use an "intelligent" forms software package. Teleform® is one example. Teleform® allows the user to create a form using multiple data collection formats. The data collection formats include multiple choice (bubbles), constrained fill-ins, and unconstrained fill-ins (handwriting or graphics). Once the form is constructed, the Teleform® software can then be used to read completed forms using multiple optical-character-recognition engines. Once the data are read, Teleform® feeds the data to multiple database formats. Because a paper form must be read, a scanner or fax machine is required. These devices communicate to a computer via direct connection or fax-modem. The disadvantage to this method is that it is necessary to learn to use the Teleform® software. The advantages are significant. This method requires relatively little equipment—resulting in reduced expense, increased equipment reliability, and decreased training requirements for data collection personnel.

COMPUTER ASSISTANCE

Computer support is very important to successful research. While many functions can be done manually, this is not the most efficient use of the researcher's time. The researcher can use the computer to

- perform literature searches
- write and revise research protocols
- correspond to sponsors, subjects, and other researchers
- develop consent forms
- test consent forms for reading and educational level to enhance subject understanding
- translate consent forms to multiple languages
- develop educational materials
- collect data
- analyze data
- perform statistical analysis
- report data

PUBLIC DOMAIN LITERATURE

There are many sources of public domain literature to assist the researcher in preparing research protocols and conducting research. The richest source of public domain literature is the Internet. Public domain literature and software are free and open to use by anyone. The Internet was originally developed by the U.S. Department of Defense and major universities to facilitate the exchange of research information. A number of search tools are available to the Internet user. Some of the better sites where searches can be done are

- Lycos—http://www.lycos.com
- Yahoo—http://www.yahoo.com
- Netsearch—http://www.excite.com
- Web Crawler—http://www.webcrawler.com

- Open Text—http://www.opentext.com
- Alta Vista—http://www.altavista.digital.com

Internet sites that the researcher will find helpful are

- National Library of Medicine—http://www.nlm.nih.gov
- National Institutes of Health—http://www.nih.gov
- World Health Organization—http://www.who.ch
- American Medical Association—http://www.ama-assn.org
- U.S. Department of Health and Human Services—http://www.os.dhhs.gov
- Centers for Disease Control and Prevention—http://www.cdc.gov
- American Society for Clinical Nutrition—http://www.faseb.org.ascn
- Dietetics Online—http://www.dietetics.com
- University of Illinois at Chicago (UIC) Library of Health Sciences—http://www.uic.edu/depts/lib/health/ahp/nmd.html
- Food and Drug Administration—http://www.fda.gov

SUMMARY

The investigator must meet numerous professional obligations. Performing an investigation that satisfies scientific, ethical, and legal requirements requires a great deal of planning. The investigator should use resources such as computer support and public domain literature and databases in planning the research. Thorough planning and recordkeeping ensures that the investigator arrives at appropriate conclusions that will stand up to the scrutiny of peer review and make meaningful contributions to the medical knowledge base.

REFERENCES

1. Fortner CL. Investigational drugs in the hospital. In: TR Brown, ed. *Handbook of Institutional Pharmacy Practice*. Bethesda, MD: American Society of Hospital Pharmacists; 1992:248.
2. *Fact Sheet*. Chicago: American Medical Association; 1994.
3. Title 21, *Code of Federal Regulations*, 50.
4. Title 21, *Code of Federal Regulations*, 50.25.
5. Title 45, *Code of Federal Regulations*, 46.

6. Food and Drug Administration. *Informed Consent and the Clinical Investigator* [Internet document: http://www.fda.gov/oc/oha/informed.html]. Washington, DC: U.S. Department of Health and Human Services; 1996.

7. Title 21, *Code of Federal Regulations*, 56.

8. *Guide for the Care and Use of Laboratory Animals.* Bethesda, MD: National Institutes of Health; 1985. U.S. Dept of Health and Human Services publication NIH 85-23.

9. Title 21, *Code of Federal Regulations*, 312.

10. Title 21, *Code of Federal Regulations*, 812.

PART II

Case Studies

CHAPTER 10

Nurse-Led Research

Marsha Evans-Orr

INTRODUCTION

Nursing research is the study of clinically relevant problems.[1] The development of the research problem in nursing does not differ from the steps used by other disciplines, and nurses often participate in interdisciplinary projects. Perhaps unique to the body of nursing research—as compared to pharmacist, physician, or dietitian research compilations—is the emphasis in published nursing research on sociological, psychological, and phenomenological research. The National Institute for Nursing Research (NINR) was founded in 1987. Originally called the National Center for Nursing Research, the organization changed its name to NINR in 1993. The NINR has focused upon nursing research using the principles of biological sciences.[2]

The nursing research presented in scholarly journals (such as *Image* and *Nursing Research*) tends to focus upon psychological, conceptual, and theoretical issues, such as perception, coping, and exploration of nursing models. Clinical practice journals (such as *Heart and Lung* or the *Journal of Parenteral and Enteral Nutrition*) tend to present physiologically based research studies led by nurses or with nurses as interdisciplinary team members. Recently, there has been an increased focus upon outcomes research in all health care disciplines, including nursing.

The American Society for Parenteral and Enteral Nutrition's "Standards of Practice: Nutrition Support"[3] identify participation in research studies and the dissemination of research findings as an essential component of the role of the nutrition support nurse. Other nursing organizations, such as the American Nurses Association, Sigma Theta Tau, and the American Organization of Nurse Executives, include statements about the evaluation of research findings and research activities within their standards of practice.[4]

To illustrate the breadth and scope of nursing research, four case studies are presented below. The case studies present examples of nurse-led, published research and summarize the materials, methods, findings, conclusions, and contributions to nursing practice. Future research to build upon findings is suggested. The examples illustrate nursing research in the physiological, technological, phenomenological (cost analysis), and psychosocial realms.

PHYSIOLOGICAL STUDY

The traditional method of initiating parenteral nutrition (PN) has been to begin at a slow administration rate and gradually increase the rate, over a period of hours or days, to a maximum infusion rate that provides appropriate kilocalories. Conversely, when PN is discontinued, current practice is to taper the rate over a period of minutes or hours before the infusion is stopped. The rationale for this practice is that insulin production increases during PN administration and decreases when PN is discontinued. Although the physiological effect of abrupt discontinuation or initiation of PN has not been well studied, clinicians fear that this practice would lead to the patient's experiencing hypoglycemia or hyperglycemia. The practice of tapering PN during initiation and discontinuation requires increased complexity in physicians' orders for PN, more time for nurses to make administration rate adjustments, and more complex infusion pump technology in the home care setting where tapering protocols for home parenteral nutrition (HPN) patients are standard practice. Although studies have reported an increase in plasma glucose during administration of PN and a decrease when it is discontinued, few have analyzed the effect of abrupt initiation or discontinuation. Kryzwda and colleagues studied plasma glucose levels during initiation and discontinuation of PN without a tapering of administration rates.[5]

Methods and Procedures

In a group of 18 patients, peripheral plasma blood glucose specimens were obtained every 5 minutes from 10 minutes prior to initiation to 120 minutes after initiation of a standard PN solution at a kilocalorie level of 1.2 times the patient's calculated resting energy expenditure. After at least 1 week of PN, the patient's blood glucose was measured before and after abrupt discontinuation of PN in the same time sequence as for the initiation of PN. The patients were also assessed for clinical signs and symptoms of hypoglycemia or hyperglycemia.

Findings and Conclusions

In this group of patients, six of whom had diabetes and three of whom were insulin-dependent, there were no clinical symptoms of hypoglycemia or hyperglycemia. During initiation, patients demonstrated a mean increase in plasma glucose of 60 mg/dL. The increase did not correlate with the amount of glucose administered. Although the mean glucose levels of patients with diabetes increased to a level that was higher than the mean of patients who were not diabetic, the difference in mean values was not significant.

The investigators concluded that use of a PN solution that provides calories at the level used in the study allows PN to be started and stopped abruptly without adverse effects. The authors stated, as a limitation, that glucose concentrations greater than those used in the study may result in responses that are different from the population in this study.

Ensuring that the sample population is large enough to avoid the error of not detecting a difference when one exists is a problem that plagues many studies in a single institution. Multicenter trials, which are more frequently seen in physician-led research than in nurse-led research, offer the advantage of increasing the sample size and, thus, avoiding a type-II error. Bendorf and colleagues demonstrated that different populations can produce different results.[6] In this study, abrupt discontinuations of PN produced hypoglycemia in 55% of the patients who were less than 3 years of age. Even tapering over 1 hour did not always prevent hypoglycemia in this age group. Further research on tapering regimens and abrupt discontinuation of PN for various age groups seems warranted.

TECHNIQUES AND PROCEDURES STUDY

Most nursing textbooks and nursing procedures require the nurse to check feeding tubes for correct placement before beginning enteral feedings or between feedings. However, techniques for assessing placement are notoriously unreliable. In fact, researchers have found that nearly all methods commonly used by nurses to assess placement of small-bore feeding tubes fail to differentiate between pulmonary and enteric placement. Installation of enteral feeding into the pulmonary system can have significant adverse consequences, including death. Thus, determining correct placement of the feeding tube is extremely important.

Metheny et al.[7] studied visual characteristics of aspirates from feeding tubes to determine whether these characteristics could be used to predict tube location accurately.

Methods and Procedures

Fluid was aspirated from 880 nasally placed feeding tubes. The samples were visually inspected and assigned one of six color labels—green, yellow or bile, off-white or tan, bloody or brown, colorless, and other. The investigators photographed 106 aspirates, and the resulting coded photographs were reviewed by a group of 30 registered nurses. The nurses were asked to predict tube placement location on the basis of the color and appearance of the aspirates. After the nurses reviewed a list of suggested visual characteristics of feeding aspirates based upon the researchers' analysis of the 880 aspirates, the nurses were asked to review the same coded photographs and, once again, predict location of the feeding tube.

Findings and Conclusions

Investigators and nurses were unable to differentiate clearly between gastrointestinal and pulmonary placement of feeding tubes based solely on visual characteristics. The nurses could detect gastric versus intestinal placement of tubes but could not reliably differentiate pulmonary from gastrointestinal placement based upon visual characteristics.

Metheny and coauthors concluded that visual characteristics are not a reliable way to determine tube placement. Their study establishes that a common practice to determine placement can lead to inaccurate results. The technique of visual inspection may be effective, however, when combined with other techniques, such as the measurement of pH. Metheny identified the study's limitations as the use of photographs rather than actual samples, possible distortion of actual color in the photographs, and overlapping criteria generated by the researchers to describe visual characteristics.

During the past decade, Metheny has studied a wide variety of methods used to test feeding tube placement. Although an ideal method has not yet been identified, Metheny's contribution to the body of nursing science in this area is substantial. Her work illustrates the power of building new research projects upon previous findings, a practice that does not occur frequently enough in nursing research.

COST-ANALYSIS STUDY

In every health care setting, there is an emphasis upon determining the cost of services and identifying essential functions. As reimbursement for services moves from heavily discounted fee-for-service to per diem to capitation agreements, clinicians must clearly understand the overall costs associated with care. Improving efficiency and reducing costs cannot be achieved without first understanding the human resources and the indirect costs required for specific therapies.

Curtas and colleagues completed an interdisciplinary analysis of the resources required for interface between home care providers and the hospital nutrition support team.[8] This descriptive study had as its stated goal to "assess the non-reimbursed costs incurred during the management of patients receiving [home parenteral nutrition]."[8]

Methods and Procedures

The investigators compiled data relating to three major resources that contribute to cost: space, furnishings, and labor costs. Space and furnishing costs were computed using depreciation, utilities, maintenance, and other expenses. Although inclusion of space and furnishing is standard business practice in out-of-hospital cost calculations used to determine fee schedules, such costs have not routinely been included in hospital-based service cost analyses. Also, in the hospital setting, labor costs are often hidden within daily room rates and are not broken out into specific clinical costs. Curtas and colleagues determined labor costs by having each member of the nutrition support team complete a time study to determine the total time spent per patient per day.[8]

Findings and Conclusions

Curtas reported a significant cost of $648 per patient per day for the hospital nutrition support team's management of home nutrition patients. These costs are in addition to those provided by home health care personnel, whose costs include labor (nurse, pharmacist, dietitian), delivery, supplies, pharmaceuticals, and indirect costs. Patient management by the primary care physician and the physician's office staff was an additional cost for some patients.

The investigators concluded that all costs should be considered when determining fair and appropriate reimbursement strategies. This interdisciplinary study demonstrates the contribution of each member of the nutrition support team to management of HPN patients. Follow-up studies might explore various models for home patient management for comparison of cost-effectiveness, resource utilization, interface among the hospital-based team and other care providers, and the effect of different management models upon patient outcome.

PSYCHOSOCIAL STUDY

With the advent of diagnosis-related groups and growth of managed care, the length of a patient's hospital stay per given diagnosis has decreased significantly during the past decade. Patients who are admitted to the hospital often leave earlier in their recovery process than they would have 10 years ago. One such example is the discharge of women within 24 hours of giving birth. Early discharge after childbirth has become standard practice in hospitals across the United States, but this practice is not without controversy.

Shorter hospital stays do not necessarily mean that significantly less care is provided. Nurses have documented that shorter lengths of stay result in a compression of activities within the new time frame. However, once the patient is discharged, the patient's family or support system bears the burden and responsibility of continuing care. The effect of shorter hospital stays upon caregivers is a prime area for nursing research, because nurses often provide services at home. Although the patient may receive other services (such as physical therapy, occupational therapy, speech therapy, or home health aide service), skilled nursing is the most common home care service.

In a descriptive study of patients' and nurses' perceptions following hospital discharge, Reiley et al explored how well nurses could predict their patients' functional ability and understanding of medications after discharge and whether patients agreed with the nurses' perceptions.[9]

Methods and Procedures

Hospitalized patients were asked to participate in a series of interviews conducted at the time of their admission, 2 weeks after hospital discharge, and 2 months after hospital discharge. The primary nurse for each patient enrolled in the study was contacted after the patient's discharge (within 2 weeks for all patients and usually within 48 hours). The investigators designed a telephone interview instrument for the nurses' interviews. They compared nurses' predictions of patients' functional status with patients' reports at the 2-month interview. Other questions from the tools used in the patients' interviews were also incorporated into the nurses' interviews. The sample population consisted of 97 nurse-patient pairs.

Findings and Conclusions

Data analysis techniques were used in this descriptive study to determine whether differences between nurses' and patients' responses were significant. The investigators found the following: nurses overestimated their patients' functional disability; there was a high level of agreement between patients' perceptions of their understanding of medications and the nurses' perceptions of the patients' understanding but significant differences in patients' and nurses' perceptions of the understanding of medication side effects; nurses overestimated patients' understanding of when to resume normal activities; and nurses overestimated patients' perceptions of the time spent preparing them for discharge.

This study demonstrates, as have others, that there is sometimes a wide gulf between the caregiver's and the patient's perceptions of patient understanding. Hospital and home care procedures typically emphasize the patient's involvement in the plan of care. This study points out that nurses must validate perceptions in order to understand where the patient's perceptions differ from the nurse's. Follow-up studies might explore the differing perceptions in specific patient populations (for example, by diagnosis, age group, or setting), after using various instructional methods or nursing interventions.

USE AND DISSEMINATION OF RESEARCH FINDINGS

Research is intended to augment and enhance the body of knowledge in a clinical area. Research findings that are not incorporated into practice do little to advance nursing science.

Cronenwett[10] has identified the following methods by which nursing research may be disseminated: literature searches, research reviews such as those provided by the Agency for Health Care Policy and Research, research conferences, and conceptual models. This author challenges clinicians to identify studies that relate to their practice, evaluate the validity of the research, develop new protocols that incorporate the research, and determine whether the protocol accomplishes the desired outcome. Although incorporation of research findings into clinical practice to advance nursing science is a laudable goal, nurses are cautioned to avoid incorporation of findings without adequate scientific evidence.

In a recent editorial on interpretation of research findings, Downs cautioned nurses to remain patient. In her words: "Researchers must be freed from pressure to jump to premature conclusions about the applications of their work. Applications will become clear in time."[11]

REFERENCES

1. Heitkemper M. Research in enteral and parenteral nutrition. In: Hennessy KA, Orr ME, eds. *Nutrition Support Nursing Core Curriculum*, 3rd ed. Silver Spring, MD: American Society for Parenteral and Enteral Nutrition; 1996:27-1–27-5.
2. Sigmon HD, Amende LM, Grady PA. Development of biological studies to support biobehavioral research at the National Institute of Nursing Research. *Image*. 1996;28:88. Guest commentary.

3. ASPEN Board of Directors. Standards of practice: nutrition support. *Nutr Clin Pract.* 1996;11:127–134.

4. Butcher LA. Research utilization in small, rural community hospital. *Nurs Clin North Am.* 1995;30:439.

5. Kryzwda EA, Andris DA, Whipple JK, Street CC, et al. Glucose response to abrupt initiation and discontinuation of total parenteral nutrition. *J Parenteral and Enteral Nutr.* 1993;27:64–67.

6. Bendorf K, Friesen CA, Roberts CC. Glucose response to discontinuation of parenteral nutrition in patients less than 3 years of age. *J Parenteral and Enteral Nutr.* 1996;20:120–122.

7. Metheny N, Reed L, Berglund B, Wehrle MA. Visual characteristics of aspirates from feeding tubes as method for predicting tube location. *Nurs Res.* 1994;43:282–287.

8. Curtas S, Hariri R, Steiger E. Case management in home total parenteral nutrition: A cost identification analysis. *J Parenteral and Enteral Nutr.* 1996;20:113–119.

9. Reiley P, Iezzoni LI, Phillips R, Davis RB, et al. Discharge planning: Comparison of patients' and nurses' perceptions of patient following hospital discharge. *Image.* 1996;28:143–147.

10. Cronenwett LR. Effective methods for disseminating research findings to nurses in practice. *Nurs Clin North Am.* 1995;30:429–437.

11. Downs FS. On clinical interpretations of research findings. *Nurs Res.* 1996;45:195. Editorial.

CHAPTER 11

Pharmacist-Led Research

Todd W. Canada and Gordon S. Sacks

INTRODUCTION

The purpose of this chapter is to examine the role of the pharmacist in conducting and participating in clinical research. This chapter discusses a research project with emphasis on specific items of importance to any health care professional involved in a clinical investigation. Funding-related issues are addressed, highlighting a multidisciplinary approach. Statistical design and analysis in a research project are described, as well as the final component of a research project—the publication. This chapter provides the reader with encouragement and a basic understanding of what is necessary to develop and implement a research idea.

ADVANCES IN PHARMACEUTICAL EDUCATION

Nutrition and drug-related research continues to evolve, with physicians, nurses, and dietitians providing important advances from their clinical experiences. The emergence of advanced entry-level and post-graduate degrees in the pharmacy profession has also enabled pharmacists to pursue these types of research. After such programs, clinical and practical training in research typically starts in specialty residencies and fellowships, with advanced pharmacy practitioners or physicians as mentors. Clinical research continues as advanced pharmacy practitioners train and integrate the residents and fellows into academic affiliations and multidisciplinary health care teams throughout the country. New pharmacy practitioners use the research skills gained from these experiences to investigate new concepts and management in nutrition support and drug therapy. This system of progression is unique because of the continued support and collaboration from advanced pharmacy practitioners after the initial training.

Only approximately 10% to 15% of U.S. pharmacists complete the training described above. How can the individuals who do not complete this specialized training learn about clinical research and have the opportunity to become involved in it? Many pharmacists are exposed to scientific research when investigational drugs are used within their health care settings. Another important way for pharmacists to gain exposure is through their involvement in various pharmacy organizations. The American Society of Health-System Pharmacists (ASHP) has provided statements and guidelines related to pharmaceutical research to encourage systematic problem solving in pharmaceutical care.[1,2] ASHP has identified several primary research areas for pharmacists because of their expertise and knowledge related to drugs. These areas include drug therapy, pharmaceutics, bioavailability, pharmacokinetics, and delivery systems. ASHP also encourages pharmacists with a research problem to seek the advice of scientific experts, such as college faculty, other staff and departments within or outside the health care setting, and individuals within the pharmaceutical industry. The American College of Clinical Pharmacy is another organization that helps pharmacists gain knowledge related to research. Both of these professional organizations have annual meetings to provide a forum for research and information exchanges. They also provide financial incentives for individuals with exceptional research projects through new investigator awards. With the exposure from job-related experiences and pharmaceutical organizations, pharmacists with the desire to become involved in research can provide critical contributions.

Although most pharmacists do not publish innovative research projects in their professional career, several pharmacists have mastered the art of research and accomplished this goal. Dickerson[3] cited numerous contributions from pharmacists that have changed clinical practices in the field of nutrition support; unfortunately, the number of these contributions has declined during the last 10 years. Obviously, funding for such research problems is becoming more difficult, and health care reform does not support research activities dramatically. However, pharmacists must not forget that the most important aspect of research is its contribution to improved patient care.

GETTING STARTED

Management-related issues specific to a particular patient population may help potential researchers develop research ideas. For pharmacists, drug-related issues are of major interest.

We identified hypomagnesemia (deficiency of magnesium [Mg] in the blood) as a common problem in the trauma intensive care unit patient population. The influence of alcohol and its close association to trauma and Mg depletion also supported this research topic. Our definition and treatment of hypomagnesemia was based upon serum Mg concentrations. However, serum Mg has not been shown to reflect the body's composition of Mg (intracellular Mg) accurately. Consequently, a protocol was developed to evaluate a new method of determining intracellular Mg concentrations. The protocol was designed to determine whether the Mg content of mononuclear blood cells (reflecting intracellular Mg concentrations) could be used to assess the efficacy of a Mg replacement regimen in critically ill, hypomagnesemic patients. This new method was compared to the conventional technique using serum Mg concentrations.

Before implementing a research protocol involving human subjects, a protocol must first be reviewed by an institutional review board (see Chapter 9). This review process protects the rights of patients and guarantees safe medical practices. We began patient recruitment only after obtaining approval from the institutional review board. This prospective clinical study was performed on consecutive patients admitted to the level-1 trauma intensive care unit with a serum Mg concentration ≤ 1.5 mg/dL. The hospital's chemistry department was asked to identify patients with a serum Mg concentration ≤ 1.5 mg/dL on a daily basis; this information was provided to the pharmacy each morning from the hospital computer system. Patients identified were screened for inclusion and exclusion criteria. In designing any study, it is important to identify variables unrelated to the intervention that may change the outcome. Many patient groups were excluded because of factors that could have confounded the interpretation of intracellular and extracellular Mg concentrations. For example, because Mg is primarily regulated by the kidney, patients with renal disease had to be excluded from study entry. For this subset of patients, it would be difficult to know whether changes in Mg concentrations were due to replacement therapy or to impaired renal function. Other exclusion criteria included patients with actual body weight $\geq 130\%$ of their ideal body weight, patients less than 18 years of age, patients who were pregnant, and patients who were seropositive for human immunodeficiency virus. If a patient met inclusion criteria, informed consent was obtained from the patient or the closest relative. The informed consent process involves a description of the research protocol, including a disclosure of any risks associated with the intervention. For example, patients were informed that Mg infusions could be associated with hypotension. However, this decrease in blood pressure could be easily treated with additional intravenous fluids. Typically, patients were identified at approximately 7:30 to 8:00 each morning from the lab report and screened before the 9:00 AM scheduled visiting hours. After the patient's family was identified and visiting hours were over, we approached the family for informed consent if the patient was unable to give consent. It took approximately 2 to 3 hours to complete this process for each patient.

The definitions of hypomagnesemia were stratified, based upon the patient's serum Mg concentration at study admission. Moderate and severe hypomagnesemia were defined as 1.1–1.5 mg/dL and ≤ 1.0 mg/dL, respectively. Depending on the degree of moderate or severe hypomagnesemia, patients received 1.0 or 1.5 mEq/kg of intravenous magnesium sulfate ($MgSO_4$), respectively. These doses were not chosen randomly, but based upon previous reports in the literature suggesting that Mg deficiency was associated with a deficit of 1 to 2 mEq/kg body weight. The dose of $MgSO_4$ was administered intravenously over 24 hours and did not exceed 8 mEq/hr. We prepared and labeled the doses within the sterile products formulation area of the pharmacy and delivered the product to the nurse for administration. It took approximately 15 to 30 minutes to complete this process for each patient.

Blood samples (20 mL) were drawn either centrally or peripherally from patients at study entry, following $MgSO_4$ infusion, and 12 and 24 hours after Mg replacement therapy. Approximately half of the blood sample was used for analysis of serum Mg, phosphorus, calcium, sodium, potassium, blood urea nitrogen, creatinine, glucose, and albumin concentrations. The serum concentrations of electrolytes other than Mg were monitored for specific reasons. Mg deficiency has been associated with a number of metabolic disorders, including hypokalemia, hypocalcemia, hypophosphatemia, and hyponatremia. From a clinician's perspective, it is important to know whether Mg deficiency is responsible for these electrolyte abnormalities. For example, if patients are hypokalemic or hypocalcemic secondary to Mg deficiency, Mg stores must be repleted first. It is well known that hypomagnesemic patients who are hypokalemic are resistant to potassium supplementation until Mg has been repleted. Mg deficiency may also cause hypocalcemia secondary to impaired secretion of parathyroid hormone. Thus, we believed that it would be beneficial to assess the relationship between intracellular Mg repletion and correction of calcium and potassium abnormalities. Obviously, blood urea nitrogen and creatinine must be monitored in order to rule out any influence of impaired renal function on Mg homeostasis. Serum glucose concentrations were observed, because glucose may induce an osmotic diuresis and cause large amounts of Mg to be lost in the urine, thereby confounding attempts to replace intracellular Mg stores. Finally, because Mg is known to be 25% bound to albumin, substantial changes in albumin concentrations may contribute to changes in serum Mg concentrations. Because monitoring these electrolytes is considered standard procedure for the trauma intensive care unit, the chemistry department of the hospital performed these analyses. The remaining portion of blood was used for determination of the intracellular Mg content. Fortunately, the nutrition support team medical director had his own laboratory adjacent to the hospital at the medical school. Intracellular Mg determinations were performed in this laboratory, and a medical technologist provided technical assistance with the Mg assay. The procedure for the determination of the intracellular Mg content was very tedious and time-consuming. Almost 2 months were required to refine this technique in order to achieve accurate intracellular Mg determinations. We discovered that the published procedure for intracellular Mg concentrations used a specific media to wash lymphocytes that was actually contaminated with Mg; thus, our laboratory values for intracellular Mg concentrations were skewed in comparison to values established in the literature. Only after testing each medium used in the analytical procedure were we able to identify and correct this problem. After several experiments, we identified an uncontaminated medium that could be used to achieve the same results. A total time of 3 to 4 hours was required to process a single blood sample from a patient.

Four blood samples were collected for each patient during the study; thus, the total lab time was 12 to 16 hours per patient.

Patient demographics, admitting diagnoses, and past medical history were obtained at the initial study assessment. Patients were also monitored daily for vital signs, electrocardiographic changes, serum laboratory values, and concurrent administration of any medications that could influence Mg homeostasis. This was accomplished with a simple monitoring form designed by one of the investigators. It took approximately 15 to 30 minutes to complete this process for each patient daily.

Approximately 12 to 16 hours per patient were required to complete the process of patient evaluation, informed consent, drug preparation, venipuncture, laboratory determination, and daily monitoring. The blood sampling also required a return trip to the hospital (usually at 9:00 to 11:00 PM) for the 12-hour post-Mg replacement collection. The time required to develop an informed consent and daily monitoring form took approximately 2 to 3 hours. The total investment of time into a research project often exceeds the traditional 8- to 10-hour workday and requires a genuine commitment to completion.

FUNDING

As with any research project, funding is always an important consideration (see Chapter 5). Financial support for this project was provided by the nutrition support team medical director. This individual has been engaged in laboratory and clinical research for 15 years and has secured numerous research grants during this time. Funds generated from large, randomized, clinical trials are frequently used to support smaller pilot studies, as was the case with this particular study. Because this was a collaborative effort between the surgery and clinical pharmacy departments, pharmacists involved in the project were granted access to laboratory space and major research equipment located in the surgery department. With regard to salary support, several of the national pharmacy and nutrition organizations offer stipends for young researchers to "start" their professional development. Most of the stipends are part of a highly competitive application process because of difficulty in obtaining funding from other traditional sources, such as industry. Fortunately, one of the authors (GS) obtained an ASHP fellowship. The other author (TC) was supported with university and hospital funding for a specialty residency in critical care and nutrition support. Without this assistance, this research project would not have been possible. The nutrition support team medical director offered support by providing lab space and resources to measure the intracellular Mg concentrations.

STUDY DESIGN AND STATISTICAL ANALYSIS

Proper study design and appropriate data analysis are critical components of a research proposal. Numerous trials have failed to demonstrate significant clinical findings solely due to flaws in study design or inappropriate statistical analysis techniques. Medical studies may be separated into two broad categories: experimental and observational studies. This particular study design is classified as an experimental study because it involved an intervention—intravenous Mg supplementation. Although a randomized, double-blind, placebo-controlled study is the most powerful study design, we chose not to use this design for a number of reasons. Our research question involved the use of a new procedure (intracellular Mg concentrations) to evaluate the efficacy of a Mg supplementation regimen. Because we were not comparing one treatment regimen to another, it was not necessary to assign patients randomly to treatment groups in order to avoid bias. Furthermore, blinding the patients and investigators to the Mg therapy was unnecessary, since the outcomes were objective determinations (intracellular and extracellular Mg concentrations). A potential weakness of the study design is the lack of a control group. In the purest sense, the best control population would have been comparable critically ill, hypomagnesemic patients who were not supplemented with intravenous Mg. However, we considered it unethical to withhold replacement therapy from critically ill, hypomagnesemic patients. Instead, we used blood samples from a group of healthy volunteers to establish a reference interval for intracellular and extracellular Mg concentrations. We then evaluated Mg concentrations to determine if therapy had normalized intracellular and extracellular Mg concentrations in the patients compared to concentrations found in the healthy volunteers.

An accurate determination of statistical power (also referred to as power analysis) is essential in a well-designed study. Conducting a power analysis reveals the ability of a study to detect the actual effect of an intervention. Thus, a study with a high power has a better chance of detecting a true difference than a study with a low power. Frequently, studies with low power indicate that the sample size is too small to detect a difference. Because our proposal was a pilot study, power calculations were not conducted *a priori* to determine adequate sample size. The dose of Mg used in our study increased serum Mg concentrations but did not significantly change intracellular Mg concentrations in the group of critically ill, hypomagnesemic patients studied. Inadequate sample size may have accounted for this observation. Post hoc calculations revealed that, in order to detect a 25% change in intracellular Mg concentrations, 41 patients would have been required to have an 80% chance of detecting a true difference. Our research project enrolled 10 patients. The limitation of small sample size is an obvious concern for this project and will be addressed in our future trials investigating this research question.

PROBLEMS ENCOUNTERED

Most research efforts unfortunately result in more questions than answers. We found serum Mg concentrations increased as expected with supplementation; however, the intracellular Mg concentrations did not reflect supplementation. The problem we encountered is probably the result of poor understanding or characterization of Mg homeostasis in the trauma patient population. Our project was designed to answer a simple question and failed to do so with our limited study group. Could we have foreseen the results of our study without pursuing it? Unfortunately, funding and time commitment are major issues when a research question requires the study of large groups of patients to show a statistical difference. The questions that emerged after our project soon may become the focus of future research by other investigators.

Original research in any field is difficult in today's health care environment. Ideally, researchers all pursue research interests with predictable conclusions. When the conclusions are not as expected, this outcome adds intrigue and frustration and points to the need for further study of the subject. After reanalyzing this project, we have identified the procedure necessary for determination of an intracellular Mg concentration. Will it give us information that will be interpretable or clinically relevant? These are the questions that must be answered to improve patient care and laboratory utilization in our current health care system.

PUBLICATION

After spending time recruiting, enrolling, studying, and evaluating patients, the most rewarding aspect of this process is publishing the results of scientific research. A peer-reviewed journal is the most prestigious place to publish, because the review process ensures quality and impartiality. Identifying the most appropriate journal often depends upon the audience that the researcher wants to reach. We submitted our manuscript to a journal that had previously published Mg-related papers. We believed that our research would make a significant contribution to the literature already published on Mg by this journal. This particular journal was affiliated with many international societies of parenteral and enteral nutrition, an audience that would be particularly interested in these results. The journal review process typically takes 6 to 12 months, and several revisions may occur before actual publication. We are currently in the second revision of this paper, 9 months after the submission of the original manuscript. The positive aspects of publishing a manuscript in a quality journal include receiving constructive comments on writing and research design, and suggestions for improvement. This experience enhances the author's writing ability and provides insight into the research methods used. Recognition of research through publication can be an important stimulus for continued personal and professional development.

SUMMARY

Clinical research is a rewarding aspect of professional development and job satisfaction. Becoming actively involved in any of the national pharmacy organizations can help facilitate an individual's research potential. Deciding on a practical and simple research project is the best method for successful completion with minimal funding and time commitment. The process of patient recruitment and consent with data collection necessitates meticulous detail for quality research. Once the research project is completed, publication of the manuscript requires professional writing skills and careful analysis. In today's changing health care environment, studies that provide data on improved patient care, improved outcomes, and decreased costs will probably be the primary recipients of funded research. The ability to design and perform research of this magnitude typically requires collaboration with experts in the field. Motivation, diligence, and commitment will enhance the person's potential for securing funded research and enable that individual to become an independent researcher in the field of clinical nutrition or pharmaceutical care.

REFERENCES

1. American Society of Hospital Pharmacists. ASHP statement on pharmaceutical research in organized health-care settings. *Am J Hosp Pharm.* 1991;48:1781.
2. American Society of Hospital Pharmacists. ASHP guidelines for pharmaceutical research in organized health-care settings. *Am J Hosp Pharm.* 1989;46:129–130.
3. Dickerson RN. Pharmacists' contribution to clinical practice through nutrition research. *Hosp Pharm.* 1996;31:1492–1496.

CHAPTER 12

Dietitian-Led Research

Jeanette M. Hasse

Elaine Monsen stated, "The strength of a discipline, whether in health sciences or management, is associated closely with its research base. Strong research supports a strong profession."[1(p 1047)] As dietitians, we want to strengthen our profession, but to many, the thought of conducting research is overwhelming. Many dietitians are apprehensive about research because they believe that research is complex, that it is reserved only for those with advanced degrees, or that there are no opportunities for research in their current positions. These myths must be dispelled in order to advance research among dietitians and other health care professions. This chapter discusses developing research ideas, implementing research studies, and the difficulties that can occur.

DISPELLING MYTHS ABOUT RESEARCH

First, the concept of research is quite elementary. It is simply asking a question and finding an answer. Dietitians conduct research every day. For example, a person who wants to go to a movie with friends asks them what movies they want to see and they indicate their choices. The person collates the results, makes a decision, and they go to a movie. This is research! The person asked a question, used a survey method to research the question, found the answer, and applied the results. A survey is one type of research that can be done. Other chapters in this book describe the types of research that can be done. To get started in research, the novice may want to begin with a simple type of research design such as a survey or a retrospective study. After gaining some experience, the novice can tackle more complicated types of research studies such as prospective, randomized, controlled trials.

Second, research can be done by any dietitian; it is not necessary to have an advanced degree to participate in research. However, an advanced degree gives the potential researcher an edge; completing a thesis or dissertation under the auspices of a professor provides a guided research experience. An individual who wants to participate in research but does not feel confident acting as a primary investigator can volunteer to help with a colleague's research project, helping to define the research question or participating in data collection.[2] After gaining some research experience, the new researcher can venture out on his or her own.

Finally, many people may think of research only as an activity done by a scientist and a handful of assistants using test tubes and bubbling liquids in a well-funded laboratory. Basic science research is very important, but clinical research is also important and is usually more practical for dietitians. However, do not assume that clinical research is easier than basic science research. There are many factors that one cannot control in a clinical research study that can make it more difficult than basic science research.[3] The main requirements for research are an inquisitive, creative, and critical mind and a question to be answered.[3] Many dietitians are practicing in clinical, managerial, and corporate settings where research can be conducted. The beginner should not expect to be given salaried time to begin a research career. In reality, new researchers may have to work research into their existing time schedules, which often means time outside of the normal work week. As researchers become more accomplished and focused, they may obtain a position or funding to devote more time to research activities.

WHY BECOME INVOLVED IN RESEARCH?

There are many reasons to participate in research. One of the foremost reasons was mentioned earlier—research will strengthen our profession. It also may save our jobs. Outcomes research has proved to be a powerful tool to justify benefits of nutrition. Many dietitians like to conduct research because of curiosity; a situation in practice has raised questions and challenged us to find answers. Research involvement is another way to enhance one's professional career. Many dietitians have found that conducting research has expanded their skills, presented new challenges, and offered opportunities they did not have before. Publication and presentation of research provide recognition for work plus an opportunity to travel to conferences and network with other professionals. Just as there are many motivations to participate in research, there are many rewards.

GETTING STARTED IN RESEARCH

Once a dietitian has decided to get involved with research, where does he or she start? Other chapters in this book give step-by-step directions for the research procedure. This chapter shares some of my personal suggestions and experiences.

The first recommendation is to find a research mentor. A mentor can be a physician, a professor, another dietitian with experience conducting research, a manager, a health care professional, someone met through networking, or an instructor at school. A researcher may have several mentors to help with different aspects of a project. Choose mentors who are willing to be teachers, and remember that newcomers to research must be willing to mentor someone else in the future.

The second recommendation is to gain experience by helping an established researcher or by obtaining a job assisting another researcher.[2] Individuals who choose to begin a research career under the auspices of an established researcher should find a way to differentiate themselves and their work from the mentor's.[3] When initiating one's own research, start with small, simple projects. This will increase the chances of success with the first experience and encourage the new researcher to continue. Examples of first projects are case studies, surveys, and retrospective studies.

My first research projects were simple reliability tests and retrospective studies. Working with liver transplant patients, I realized that many of the patients I saw were malnourished; however, objective nutrition assessment measurements were invalid in patients with end-stage liver disease. A friend had shown me an article about a technique called subjective global assessment that was valid and reliable when used with other patient populations.[4] I adapted this technique for liver transplant patients and tested it for reliability (ie, could another dietitian get the same results as mine using this assessment tool?). This was my first research project.[5] Then I began to wonder "How many patients are malnourished, and does malnutrition make a difference in their posttransplant outcomes?" As are other dietitians, I am a great collector of data. I had nutrition records of several hundred transplant patients, and their medical data were stored in a computerized database within our transplant department. A statistical analysis of these data supported my hypothesis that malnutrition was prevalent among liver transplant candidates and resulted in lengthened posttransplant hospitalizations.[6] This project is an example of a simple retrospective study using data already collected. I conducted other retrospective studies to answer other questions that had developed in my practice over the years.[7,8] Finding answers to research questions usually leads to other questions. My early retrospective studies led me to the next stage of conducting prospective, randomized, controlled studies.

DEVELOPING A RESEARCH TRIAL

Prospective, randomized, controlled trials with at least one treatment group and one control group are considered to be the standards for evaluating interventions.[9,10] Prospective studies typically require more planning and effort than retrospective studies. The first prospective, randomized, controlled study I conducted was to evaluate the benefit of early postoperative enteral feeding on outcomes of patients undergoing liver transplantation.[11] The basic steps to set up a research project are outlined in Exhibit 12–1. The discussion below walks the reader through research design steps, using my experience as an example.

Selecting a Research Topic

The first step in conducting research is to select the research topic.[1] Most research studies evolve from questions that arise in our practice.[12] When selecting an area of research, it may be helpful to remember the following principles. Anticipate the results; if the most interesting outcome won't make much impact, then the project may not be worth pursuing.[3] A research topic should be relevant to practice and of significant interest to the researcher.[3,13] If the interest is the researcher's alone, he or she may have difficulty obtaining funding. On the other hand, if the profession values the research, but the researcher finds it uninteresting, he or she will have a difficult time completing the project or finding the initiative to

Exhibit 12–1 Basic Steps To Design a Research Project

1. Select a research topic.
2. Conduct a thorough literature review.
3. Define your hypothesis.
   - The hypothesis must be testable.
   - The hypothesis must be based on previous research or experiences.
4. Define your research question(s).
   - Answer who, what, and how.
5. Write a study proposal.
   - Define aims and objectives.
   - Describe the significance of your research.
   - Outline the methodology in detail.
6. Have someone review your proposal. Adjust your proposal based on those reviews.
7. Find funding for your study.
8. Obtain approval from your institutional review board or human subjects review committee.
9. Implement your study.
10. Always adhere to ethical practices.
11. Review the results of your study.
12. Present your findings.
13. Develop new research questions.

spend many hours working on it. Third, researchers should try to find a niche that is underoccupied and to create opportunities to "build on a theme."[2,3] For example, very little nutrition research was being conducted in the transplant field when I started working with transplant patients, so it was a natural topic for me to research. High-risk, high-interest research projects offer researchers an opportunity to advance in their career and make significant contributions to their field, but it is important to balance those studies with some low-risk projects.[3] I try to intersperse time-intensive prospective projects with simpler retrospective studies. Researchers should be prepared to learn new skills or invite a collaborator to participate if a project involves some expertise they do not have.[2] I have found that experts in a special technique or field of research are willing to be coinvestigators. I gain knowledge from them, and they gain experience with a new research topic or population that they would not have had without my invitation—a win-win situation.

The idea for my first prospective study, an evaluation of early postoperative feeding in liver transplant patients, stemmed from a couple of sources. First, my retrospective research had shown a dismal picture that 70% of our liver transplant patients were malnourished, which adversely affected their recovery and increased hospitalization costs.[5] Second, studies evaluating early feeding in other patient populations showed favorable results.[14,15] I wondered if early feeding would improve the outcomes of my patients. This was the basis for my prospective study evaluating the benefits of early postoperative tube feeding in liver transplant patients.

Defining the Hypothesis and Research Question

A hypothesis is a statement predicting the relationship between variables being studied within a specified population.[16] A hypothesis must be testable and have a scientific rationale based on previous research or experience.[16] An extensive literature review evaluates what has already been done and provides ideas for the researcher's project. When I was reviewing the literature for my project, there was only one nutrition support study in adult liver transplant patients, and it evaluated parenteral, not enteral, nutrition. To provide a framework for my study, I also studied literature comparing enteral feeding to other forms of nutrition in general surgical patients.

After reviewing the literature, the researcher must define the research question. To do this, the researcher must ask "Who, what, and how."[1,2] The question must be clearly stated so that others will know what the researcher is investigating.[12] My subjects ("who") were defined as patients at least 18 years of age who were undergoing liver transplantation at my institution. To keep results from being swayed by uncontrolled variables, patients with certain conditions such as renal failure and carcinoma were eliminated from the study. If the researcher wishes to stratify the subjects, this approach must be planned and stated in the proposal before the study is begun.[12] The "what" in my study consisted of the different immediate postoperative treatments to be randomly given to the patients—either tube feeding plus intravenous fluids or intravenous fluids alone. The "how" to detect differences in treatment consisted of multiple measurable outcome variables. End points must be explicitly identified and defined.[12] The variables I measured on posttransplant days 2, 4, 7, and 14 were resting energy expenditure (REE), nitrogen balance, and handgrip strength. I chose these days to represent specific time points in the posttransplant recovery phase; most patients were in the intensive care unit on day 2, transfer to the regular nursing floor usually occurred by day 4, day 7 represented the 1-week posttransplant mark, and many patients were discharged by day 14. Calorie and protein intake was measured daily for 12 posttransplant days. The incidences of infection and rejection were monitored for the first 21 days after transplantation, and the number of days on the ventilator, the number of days in intensive care, hospital lengths of stay, and hospitalization charges during the initial hospitalization were evaluated.

Writing a Study Proposal

Once the question is well defined, the researcher must write the study proposal. The first part of the protocol is the research question, also known as specific aims and objectives.[1] This step is discussed above. The second part of the proposal describes the significance of the research project. This is where the researcher convinces the supervisor, institutional review board (IRB), funding source, and whoever will be reviewing the proposal that it is worthwhile. This section must answer two basic questions: "Why is this research important?" and "Why is it unique?" Part of the rationale for my study was to determine whether enteral nutrition could improve nutritional status, decrease complication rates following liver transplantation, and enhance posttransplant recovery. The third part of the proposal should discuss previous work in this area by the particular researcher or others; this information should have been collected in the earlier literature review.

Next, the researcher should write a detailed methodology. The methodology must be clear and concise and include subject and control selection, degree of blinding, specific interventions, the research setting, what measurements will be made, who will perform the measurements, description of instruments, and how patients' rights will be protected.[10,17] I defined how patients were to be selected and randomized to the treatment groups, and I defined the process of consent. The types of treatment, either tube feeding plus intravenous fluids or intravenous, had to be carefully explained. For the treatment group, I had to decide what type of feeding tube to use, when the feeding tubes would be placed, when tube feeding would begin, what formula would be used, how the feedings would be monitored, when oral diets would be initiated, and when the tubes would be removed. It was not possible to blind the study because it was easy to see who was being tube-fed and who was not. However, in a study comparing different enteral formulas, the patient and investigators could be blinded to the intervention, provided that the formulas looked similar. In my study, the diets were advanced at the same rate for both groups. Each of the variables to be measured had to be specifically outlined. I had to define when REE, nitrogen balance, and grip strength would be measured; what equipment would be used; and who would do the measurements. I had to define infection and rejection and specify how they would be diagnosed and measured. I had to determine how I would obtain information about the amount of time each patient spent on the ventilator, in the intensive care unit, and in the hospital. I also had to determine whether I could obtain and measure hospital costs or charges.

The final part of the methodology is to choose appropriate statistical methods.[10,17] My advice is to have a professional statistician do this. A researcher whose department does not have a statistician can hire a statistician to consult; some statisticians contribute their time for coauthorship. To locate a statistician, ask a mentor for suggestions or check with local universities. I recommend taking a class in statistics or finding a good book that describes the use of statistical methods. It is not necessary to know how to run the statistical tests, but it is important to have a basic understanding of what tests are best suited to answer specific questions and how to interpret the results. A statistician will not only analyze the data but also help to determine the number of subjects necessary to determine a significant difference.

Once the proposal is written, it is important to have someone else review it. Other professionals may be able to point out improvements that the writer has not considered. Consider asking a mentor or coworker who will critically and thoughtfully review the proposal and provide feedback. I have found it helpful to have colleagues and the Dietitian's Research Support Group of the American Society for Parenteral and Enteral Nutrition critique my proposals.

Funding the Study

Once the proposal is written, the researcher must determine the budget and funding sources. When preparing a budget, it is important to consider all the costs associated with the study. Guidelines and helpful hints on preparing grant proposals are described in Chapter 5. Again, mentors can review the budget to ensure that the proposal includes all costs and that it is competitive. A sample of expense items for my tube-feeding study is listed in Exhibit 12–2.

Exhibit 12–2 Expense Items for a Study Comparing Tube-Fed to Non–Tube-Fed Liver Transplant Patients

Supplies

- feeding tubes
- tube-feeding bags and sets
- tube-feeding formulas
- grip strength dynamometer

Tests

- laboratory tests (urine urea nitrogen)
- metabolic cart studies

Personnel Costs

- dietitians' salaries
- statistician's fees
- data entry personnel fees

Miscellaneous Costs

- overhead (usually a percentage set by each institution)
- feeding tube placement fees
- duplication of forms
- slides or poster to present results at a professional meeting
- preparation of a manuscript
- travel to present research results

Be creative in obtaining funds for a study and consider several sources if one source is not adequate. I used several different sources to fund my tube-feeding study. Staff members who helped with the study donated their time, and all participants were recognized as coauthors. A nutrition company supplied tube-feeding formula, and another company donated tube-feeding containers, tubing, and pumps. The pulmonary and laboratory departments agreed to run the metabolic cart studies and laboratory tests at cost. I obtained a small grant from Dietitians in Nutrition Support Practice Group to pay for these expenses. Finally, my department paid for the statistician's time and the costs associated with travel to present the study.

Obtaining Approval

Early in the developmental phase, it is important to obtain approval for pursuing the project from one's department or director. Once the study proposal has been written and funding has been obtained, it is necessary to obtain approval from the IRB. It is imperative that studies involving human subjects be reviewed and approved by a human studies committee.[12] Researchers should contact their IRB for guidelines for approval and follow the IRB guidelines precisely. Typically, the researcher must provide a proposal, consent forms, and other specific forms describing the research and the risks and benefits of the study. When writing consent forms, avoid medical jargon and use simple language to convey the study's risks and benefits. For example, rather than stating that the study needs a 5-mL sample of blood, state that about 1 teaspoon of blood is needed. I found it helpful to ask someone who was familiar with the IRB process to help me with the forms the first time I had to complete them.

Implementing the Study

Once the proposal is approved, it is time to set up all the procedures for the study. It is necessary to plan how each step will happen and who is responsible for each step. This can be the most tedious part of research, but planning carefully will make conducting the study much easier. Once again, get help from those who have research experience to make sure nothing has been overlooked. For my tube-feeding study, I had to determine who would be responsible for each step (see Exhibit 12–3).

I took some preparatory steps to ease the implementation of my study. First, I informed and gave inservices to all personnel and departments involved in the study including surgeons, anesthesiologists, research nurses, and patient nursing and nutrition department personnel. I developed standing orders to implement the processes for the study and developed data collection forms before the study was initiated. It is easier to collect data prospectively—to gather all the information that may be necessary and then not use some of it—than it is to realize that some of the data are missing and to have to retrieve the information retrospectively. I conducted a pilot study to ensure that tube feeding as proposed for the study was tolerated by transplant recipients. With input from the statistician, I determined the number of subjects for the study as well as the format for data collection and entry. I developed a timeline and learned the importance of being realistic when determining how long it would take to

---

Exhibit 12–3 Questions I Had To Ask When Implementing a Study Evaluating the Benefits of Early Posttransplant Tube Feeding

1. Who would identify patients eligible for the study?
2. Who would contact the patients about their interest in participating in the study?
3. How would I be notified when a patient was to be transplanted?
4. Who could complete the consent process with the patients, and when would the patients participate in this process?
5. Once patients consented to participate in the study, how would they be randomized?
6. How would other team members be involved, and how would they be informed about the study?
7. Who would order the tests to be done?
8. Who would perform the tests and when?
9. How would all the departments be notified when a patient was entered into the study?
10. How would the data be collected, entered into a database, and analyzed?
11. Who would perform the statistical tests?
12. How would the charges for the study be billed to my study account?
13. How long would it take to complete this study?

complete a study. Researchers can review past records to help determine how many patients would be eligible for a study and how long it would take to reach a given sample size,[12] but there often are uncontrollable outside variables that influence the progress of the study. A flowchart outlining procedures for defining each step of the study and who is responsible for each section can be helpful (see Figure 12–1).

Adhering to Ethical Practices

It is important that researchers adhere to ethical practices in research.[2] No matter the size or complexity of a study, researchers should always follow principles of good study preparation and management. For example, previously published reports and ideas should be referenced and data should not be falsified or manipulated to obtain results that the researcher wanted or expected.

Dealing with Unforeseen Events

The culmination of the researcher's planning is entering the first subject into the study. The entry of the first few subjects is one of the most difficult and time-consuming aspects of the actual study. Preparation and careful planning should help the study run smoothly. However, no matter how well researchers plan, they always have to deal with unforeseen events. In most studies, researchers rely on many people and circumstances that they cannot control. Not only are researchers at the mercy of the subjects, but of those who help. We try to predict, as best we can, how many subjects will be available for a study. Unforeseen factors usually affect the actual enrollment into studies.

Changes in recruitment, enrollment, and dropout rates similarly affect the number of subjects in the study. Recruitment of subjects can be problematic; patients must be willing to accept the treatment in the study. The number of admitted patients who meet criteria for entry into a study can be less than what the researcher predicts. In my situation, other studies running concurrently with mine competed for subjects. We devised a strategy so that every other patient undergoing transplantation was eligible to enroll in my study. Even though there was little risk involved in the study, some patients chose not to participate. Those who do choose to par-

Primary investigator (PI) or coinvestigators identify patients eligible for the study.

↓

PI has patients complete informed consent process for study while patients are on waiting list for transplant.

↓

Research nurse notifies PI when a patient is to be transplanted.

↓

Patient admitted to hospital for transplant.

↓

PI makes sure that patient has completed informed consent process for study if not done previously.

↓

PI opens randomization envelope to identify patient group.

↓

PI notifies surgeon and anesthesiologist if feeding tube should be placed during surgery.

↓

PI or coinvestigator notifies intensive care unit (ICU) of patient's treatment group.

↓

ICU nurse or aide places standing orders for treatment in patient's medical record.

↓

Aide enters standing orders into computer.

↓

PI calls pulmonary lab to make sure metabolic cart studies are scheduled.

↓

Nurses administer tube feeding to patients in experimental group.

↓

PI or coinvestigator monitors tube feeding and keeps tube-feeding supplies in stock.

↓

PI or coinvestigator performs grip strength tests, changes rate of tube feeding, and initiates calorie counts per protocol.

↓

PI or coinvestigator collects data and orders discontinuation of feeding tube per protocol.

↓

Data entry personnel enter data into computer database.

↓

PI reviews raw data, which are forwarded to statistician.

↓

Statistician analyzes data and returns results to PI.

↓

PI and coinvestigators evaluate results and draw conclusions.

Figure 12–1 Example of a flowchart outlining responsibilities of investigators for a research study evaluating tube feeding in liver transplant recipients.

ticipate in a study may actually bias the study or affect validity because they are aware of being in a study and may alter their behavior.[18] In addition, patients often differ in their response to treatment and their participation in studies.[9] If a study relies on active patient participation, there may be a bias toward those who participate actively.

Subject dropout can occur for many reasons. Patients may move or have other legitimate reasons for withdrawing from a study, such as inability to attend scheduled appointments due to lack of transportation. However, if subjects drop out because of the treatment that they were randomly assigned, the groups cannot be regarded as being random.[4] Data from studies with large dropout rates are more difficult to evaluate than those with low dropout rates.[4] Our dropout rate was higher than anticipated; we evaluated our data on an "intent-to-treat" basis as well as on a basis of patients who actually completed the study.

Regardless of whether a research study uses an animal or human model, the people who run the tests may leave, the funding may be reduced, coinvestigators may take new jobs, or the principal investigator may have a job change. All of these factors are beyond the researcher's control. Researchers cannot predict what events will happen that will affect their studies. All they can do is to deal with each problem as soon as it arises and make adjustments without changing the study aims.

When major changes in the protocol occur or if adverse events occur, the researcher should inform the IRB. If the original timeline is not accurate, it may be necessary to contact funding sources to apply for extensions. The researcher should complete a regular evaluation of progress and the project's budget and be willing to evaluate whether to continue the study if it is not answering the research questions.

Finally, with perseverance and some good luck, the researcher will complete the study, be able to analyze the data, and answer the research questions. After successfully completing the research project, the research team should study it and think about how it could have been improved.[1] Once the researcher has analyzed results and drawn some conclusions, it is important to share those results, not only with those who helped with the study but also with those interested in the research topic. Results of my study were presented at a national nutrition meeting and were published in a journal.[11]

Finding the answers to research questions often reveals new questions that may direct the researcher to another research study. We continue to look at the impact of pre- and postoperative nutrition support on transplant outcome; we are also investigating the benefits of anabolic agents in addition to nutrition support in transplant patients. Research is infectious; after completing one study, the researcher is already thinking about the next. The advantage is that the researcher can use completed research as a guide for the next research question.[1] It is important to focus one's research on one or two project areas.[3] A researcher is more likely to make an impact in the profession if he or she is focused rather than trying to investigate several areas.

SUMMARY

Conducting research is challenging and rewarding. Anyone who has a curious mind and pays attention to detail can conduct research. Dietitians can and should be involved in nutrition research to create a strong and lasting profession.

REFERENCES

1. Monsen ER, Cheney CL. Research methods in nutrition and dietetics: Design, data analysis, and presentation. *J Am Diet Assoc.* 1988;88:1047–1065.

2. Kubena KS. Research and discovery: Getting started. *Support Line.* 1997;19(3):4–6.

3. Kahn CR. Picking a research problem—the critical decision. *N Engl J Med.* 1994;330:1530–1533.

4. Detsky AS, McLaughlin JR, Baker JP, Johnston N, et al. What is subjective global assessment of nutritional status? *J Parenteral and Enteral Nutr.* 1987;11:8–13.

5. Hasse JM, Strong S, Gorman MA, Liepa GU. Subjective global assessment: Alternative nutrition assessment technique for liver transplant candidates. *Nutrition.* 1993;9:339–343.

6. Hasse JM, Blue LS, Crippin JS, Goldstein RM, et al. The effect of nutritional status on length of stay and clinical outcomes following liver transplantation. *J Am Diet Assoc.* 1994;94(suppl):A-38. Abstract.

7. Hasse JM, Ball CA. Long-term nutritional problems in adult liver transplant recipients. *J Am Diet Assoc.* 1990;90(suppl):A-36. Abstract.

8. Hasse JM. Effect of pretransplant obesity and nutrition education on weight gain following liver transplantation. *J Am Diet Assoc.* 1992;92(suppl):A-82. Abstract.

9. Bradley C. Designing medical and educational intervention studies. *Diabetes Care.* 1993;16:509–518.

10. Haughey BP. Evaluating quantitative research designs: Part 1. *Crit Care Nurs.* 1994;14:100–102.

11. Hasse JM, Blue LS, Liepa GU, Goldstein RM, et al. Early enteral nutrition support in patients undergoing liver transplantation. *J Parenteral and Enteral Nutr.* 1995;19:437–443.

12. Twomey PL. Getting started in clinical nutrition research. *Nutr Clin Pract.* 1991;6:175–183.

13. Finnick M, Haughey BP. Evaluating quantitative research problems. *Crit Care Nurs.* 1992;12:98–105.

14. Kudsk KA, Croce MA, Fabian TC, Minard G, et al. Enteral versus parenteral feeding: Effects on septic morbidity after blunt and penetrating abdominal trauma. *Ann Surg.* 1992;215:503–513.

15. Moore FA, Feliciano DV, Andrassy RJ, McArdle AH, et al. Early enteral feeding compared with parenteral reduces postoperative septic complications: The results of a meta-analysis. *Ann Surg.* 1992;216:172–183.

16. Haughey BP. A guide to evaluating hypotheses and definitions of variables. *Crit Care Nurs.* 1992;12:98–103.

17. Peters DD. Materials and methods. *J Endodontics.* 1993;19:420–421.

18. Haughey BP. Evaluating quantitative research designs: Part 2. *Crit Care Nurs.* 1994;14:69–72.

CHAPTER 13

Physician-Led Research

Orlando C. Kirton and David V. Shatz

INTRODUCTION

Physician-led research will be increasingly important in the evolving health care environment. High-quality, cost-effective care will depend on evidence-based, data-driven, technological, pharmaceutical, and clinical outcomes studies. These outcomes studies can range from institutional, continuous quality improvement (CQI) protocols and critical care pathways to multicenter, randomized prospective clinical trials. The physician's role and accountability to ensure efficacy and effectiveness will undoubtedly increase. The physician in the role of researcher must provide multidisciplinary team leadership. The ultimate goal is the delivery of efficient, effective, high-quality care while minimizing costs.

DEFINING THE QUESTION

The physician must design the activity for monitoring or evaluating outcomes that will be both practical and beneficial to a specific patient cohort, medical/surgical service, or specialty unit. He or she must ensure that the requirements of the research endeavor are within the scope of the available resources (eg, subject accrual, materials, and financial support).

Retrospective chart reviews are useful in generating hypotheses, determining the incidence of disease occurrence, and determining expected subject availability. The published literature must be interpreted by the strength of its scientific content. This approach is called evidence-based medicine; it is based on knowledge of the evidence upon which a prac-

235

tice or hypothesis is derived and the validity of that evidence. Evidence-based analysis involves precisely defining a problem, proficiently researching it, and critically appraising and assimilating relevant information from the literature.[1] The citation level of evidence ranges from (1) randomized, prospective, controlled investigation; (2) nonrandomized investigation with concurrent or historical controls or peer-reviewed state-of-the-art articles, to (3) case series, textbook, or other such non–peer-reviewed publications.[2] Accordingly, recommendations regarding any therapeutic regimen, policy, or treatment protocol can be stratified into three levels of substantiation: (1) convincingly justifiable on scientific evidence alone; (2) reasonably justifiable by the available literature and buttressed by expert opinion; or (3) widely supported by expert opinion or available data but lacking adequate scientific evidence. Without systematic review, the researcher may miss promising leads or embark on studies whose questions have already been answered.

DEVELOPING THE RESEARCH PROTOCOL

It is important to define the hypotheses, objective(s), rationale, patient population, statistical design, sample size, and methodology. The hypothesis must state the researcher's expectations of the study result or finding; it must be significant, testable, and supported by the chosen methodology. The aim (or project objective) of the study must be focused and test the hypotheses. Preliminary background data provide the rationale for the hypotheses and demonstrate capability and feasibility. The researcher must clearly state the methodology and its rationale, minor/major violations, and primary/secondary end points. The statistical methods or design should be appropriate for the data collected. Dropout and withdrawal criteria must be considered, and statistical power assumptions should be well defined. The patient population must also be clearly defined, and entrance and exclusion criteria must be consistent. Data quality definition should include criteria for collecting, analyzing, and assessing clinical and laboratory data and defining the accuracy of the data, including intra- and interoperator biases and errors.

Clinical information systems are known by several different names, including bedside information systems, patient care systems, medical information systems, bedside charting systems, and patient charting systems. Clinical information systems automatically acquire, display, and report patient information. Integrating patient research with a clinical information system can have a positive impact on research. Capturing data electronically minimizes manual transcription and lowers the chances of transcription error. Time spent in data collection is markedly reduced, as are the person-hours and personnel required to acquire the data. These and other reduced demands make research more attractive and user-friendly.

A multidisciplinary team comprised of interested, knowledgeable individuals should compose the planning committee. It is important to include all disciplines that provide patient care into the development of research protocols and use realistic time frames associated with thorough education of the immediate staff and crucial ancillary personnel. It is essential to provide instruction about identification of adverse events and documentation of variances or deviations from the protocol.

DETERMINING THE SAMPLE SIZE

Start by entering the best estimate of the incidence rate of the disease or outcome to be studied. Does the researcher expect the test group rate to be higher or lower, and what is the smallest difference between the test group and control that the researcher wants to detect? What level of certainty is necessary to detect a difference if it truly exists (ie, beta error), and what level of certainty is necessary to determine whether any differences between the test group and control are simply due to chance (ie, alpha error)? Both the alpha and beta error are affected by the researcher's decisions. For example, given a 30% incidence rate (eg, nosocomial pneumonia), if a 15% change is considered significant (eg, the preventive strategy is effective), and given a 5% alpha error and 5% beta error, 100 patients per group would be required. If the researcher lowers expectations from 15% to a 10% difference, the sample size increases from 100 to 271 patients per group.

THE INFORMED CONSENT

Informed consent is one of the primary ethical requirements for research with human subjects. The competent patient or health care proxy has the right to choose or refuse to participate, based on the concepts of informed consent and informed refusal. The components of informed consent include (1) the provision of sufficient and accurate information from the health care provider, (2) patient comprehension, and (3) the exercise of free choice.[3] The consent must contain the following: title, purpose, procedure, known risks, benefits, alternatives, compensation, confidentiality guarantee, right to withdraw, and any other pertinent information (such as who to contact and how to reach them in case of emergencies or questions) (see Exhibit 13–1).

Exhibit 13–1 Informed Consent: Example

Title: Evaluation of a new total antioxidant status (TAS) kit in a healthy population

Introduction: You have been asked to participate in a research study to evaluate a new laboratory kit that measures the presence of antioxidants in peripheral blood (plasma).

Purpose of the research: The new kit is manufactured by Randox (Cumlin, Great Britain). The purpose of the study is: (1) to evaluate the **normal values** of antioxidants in a healthy population, and (2) to have the laboratory technicians become familiarized with the new kit.

Procedures: You will be one of the 20 individuals participating in the study. You must be healthy and a nonsmoker. Five mL of blood (a teaspoon) will be drawn from a peripheral antecubital vein. The procedure will be done by a certified nurse or physician.

Risks: The risks of blood drawing include: fainting; temporary discomfort and/or bruise at the site of puncture; and, rarely, infection or the formation of a small clot or swelling to the vein and surrounding area.

Compensation: No compensation is available if any injury occurs to you as a direct result of the blood drawing itself, beyond that provided under the direction of your doctor.

Confidentiality: Your consent to participate in this study includes consent for the investigator and his or her assistants to review all medical records as may be necessary for the purposes of the study. The investigator and assistants will consider all records confidential to the extent permitted by law. Records and results will not be identified as pertaining to you in

continues

Exhibit 13–1 continued

any publication without express permission. In rare circumstances, the U.S. Food and Drug Administration (FDA) or the U.S. Department of Health and Human Services (DHHS) may request copies of the medical records. If this happens, the FDA or DHHS requests will be granted.

Right to withdraw: Participation in this study is entirely voluntary. Refusal to participate or request for withdrawal at any time during the study is permitted without penalty or loss of any benefits to which you are otherwise entitled.

_____   _____

Patient's Signature   Date

_____   _____

Witness's Signature   Date

DATA-DRIVEN OUTCOMES ASSESSMENT

The use of strict protocols to direct care should supplement the capability of the physician to meet or exceed targeted performance standards and should not be viewed as eliminating or restricting the physician's prerogative. These protocols should be detailed, algorithm-based, and easily computerized, reducing variability to a minimum. All protocol overrides by physicians must be justified and documented, thus becoming the foundation by which the process remains dynamic and new discoveries and ideas surface. A research protocol allows evaluation of therapy, and continuous evolution of the protocol constantly reestablishes a reference baseline. Standardized protocols allow the role of a new product or policy to be defined, thus eliminating ineffective ones and strengthening the effectiveness of others. The list of common practices in which scrutiny is necessary could be endless but should contain individual preferences or the routine "protocols" in one's own unit. Two case examples are reviewed below: (1) management of paroxysmal, new-onset, supraventricular tachycardia (PSVT); and (2) catheter sepsis.

1. A prior review at our institution revealed a 3.4% incidence of PSVT during a 6-month period. With treatment left to the discretion of the physician on call, arrhythmia control with conversion occurred in only 60% of patients in 24 hours. The efficacy of a new treatment algorithm involving the sequential administration of different classes of anti-arrhythmic agents to produce conversion to normal sinus rhythm and heart rate control was evaluated. Preliminary data suggested that a multiagent algorithm, incorporating several anti-arrhythmic agents acting at different receptor sites within the atrial pacemaker and atrioventricular node provided rapid, effective control of acute-onset PSVT in 100% of patients.[4] Additionally, the pharmacological regimen had to be continued until the acute stress state abated in surgical patients.

2. Strict guidelines for the use and maintenance of central venous access catheters, pulmonary artery catheters, and arterial catheters should be based on available data specific to in-house intensive care unit (ICU) patients. If guidelines for aseptic technique and catheter maintenance are strictly adhered to, catheter-related infections can be reduced. Civetta and others demonstrated that the rate of catheter-related infections increased after the sixth ICU day in both clean and septic patients.[5] Using the technique described by Maki and colleagues,[6] guidewire exchanges of catheters and cultures of the intracutaneous segment can direct the diagnosis and treatment of catheter-related sepsis. Detailed records of catheter microbiology history are necessary to ensure that catheters are changed appropriately. Ball and colleagues[7] have shown a 28% incidence of contamination on the first exchange (mean 4.1 day), with decreasing rate of contamination of subsequent catheters exchanged over a guidewire to 6% by the fourth exchange. We recently substituted antimicrobial-impregnated, triple-lumen catheters for standard catheters in patients who required central venous access. Catheters impregnated with sulfadiazine-chlorhexidine decreased the incidence of catheter infection.[8] Chlorhexidine alters membrane permeability with the subsequent entry and binding of silver ions to the bacterial DNA helix. Protected catheters were found to have a significantly lower rate of infection (defined as a positive intracutaneous segment culture) than unprotected catheters. Also, whereas unprotected catheters had an increased rate of infection after 10 days, protected catheters did not. The ability to leave these catheters safely in position for a longer period of time reduces the risk and

expense of multiple guidewire exchanges. We found cost savings of $5000 per month in our ICU using protected catheters.

EVALUATION OF NEW TECHNOLOGY

Technological advances have not always received rigorous analysis appropriate to assess impact on the overall clinical efficacy and patient outcomes in the critical care arena (eg, pulmonary artery catheters). With the advent of health care reform, it is clear that future equipment and pharmaceuticals, which are left to market demands or governmental regulations, will have to be justified by the ability to prevent or reduce the number of complications and/or reduce the total cost. We must evaluate the "newest" forms of technology for more than potential or touted "advantages"; we must assess the personnel and time involved, because these costs are commonly thought to represent nearly 70% of hospital budgets. There is great potential to improve the efficacy of care through outcomes-based research. Our experience with minimally invasive respiratory monitoring in mechanically ventilated patients is an example of outcomes assessment for a new technology.

Portable microprocessor-based respiratory monitors such as the Bicore CP-100 (Allied Healthcare, Riverside, California) measure many parameters of mechanical ventilation and respiratory function, including compliance, airway resistance, strength and endurance, and both patient and ventilator work of breathing. Work of breathing, which is calculated as the product of the change in pressure and lung volume, is a measure of the process of overcoming the elastic and frictional forces of the lung and chest wall.[9]

We became increasingly aware of the impact of imposed work performed by the patient to breathe through the endotracheal tube, the breathing circuit, and the ventilator-demand system, contributing to apparent ventilator dependency.[10] A prospective, descriptive data collection was conducted for 1 year to evaluate the importance of tachypnea as an indicator of ventilatory failure during our usual 20-minute preextubation trial of room air, 5 cm of H_2O continuous positive airway pressure when associated with elevated imposed work of breathing.

Patients were weaned to minimal mechanical ventilatory support and underwent a preextubation trial if airway protection was likely and secretions minimal. When passed ($PaO_2 \geq 55$ torr, $PaCO_2 \leq 45$ torr with prior eucapnia, the pH of arterial blood (pHa) $\geq$ 7.35, respiratory rate $\leq$ 30 breaths/minute), extubation followed. If patients failed due to hypoxemia, ventilator support resumed. If tachypnea was the reason for failure, work of breathing was measured with the Bicore CP-100 (Allied Medical Products, Riverside, CA). If patient work of breathing was $\leq$ 1.1 joules/L, extubation proceeded despite tachypnea. If patient work of breathing > 1.1, imposed work of breathing was measured, and if resultant physiologic work of breathing (patient work of breathing - imposed work of breathing) was $\leq$ 0.8 joules/L, patients were extubated.[11] Of 589 extubations, 105 (18%) were classified as false-negatives based on a preextubation rate of > 30 breaths/minute. Of these, 97 were successfully extubated despite tachypnea ranging from 32 to 56 breaths/minute, when combined with either a patient work of breathing $\leq$ 1.1 joules/L or physiologic work of breathing $\leq$ 0.8 joules/L. The rate of extubation failure within 72 hours was 7.6% (8/105) in the tachypnea group, compared to 7.9% (38/484) for those with respiratory rates $\leq$ 30 breaths/minute. Average duration of mechanical ventilation during the study period decreased by 2 days from 8.6 to 6.3 days (p = .03).

We concluded that tachypnea as a marker of respiratory distress is sensitive but is not sufficiently specific to be used as a criterion in preextubation trials. The decrease in the duration of mechanical ventilation by 2 days in this study, while not due solely to the change in extubation criteria, has significant cost and bed-resource implications. Based on a 2-day decrease in the duration of ventilatory support, the 105 tachypneic extubations may have added between 105 and 210 "extra" critical care bed days during the year, or at the very least, one "extra" bed for 7 months.

MULTI-INSTITUTIONAL TRIALS

Participation in collaborative, multi-institutional trials may be necessary to pool resources, increase the patient pool, and add geographic diversity. However, such trials require special organizational structures to ensure the uniformity of data acquisition and quality at each clinical unit. We embarked on a prospective, randomized, double-blind, multi-institutional trial to compare a 24-hour versus a 5-day course of a single broad-spectrum antibiotic for penetrating abdominal trauma with associated hollow viscus gastrointestinal injury. There is compelling evidence supporting that a short course of perioperative antibiotics is safe and effective; however, previous studies suffered from inadequate stratification, lack of standardized approaches to irrigation of the peritoneum and management of wounds, and lack of standardization in the antibiotic agent administered. Primary end points of our protocol included wound and intraabdominal infections. Secondary end points included the incidence of urinary tract infections, pneumonia, bacteremia, and cellulitis. A threshold criteria to unblind a study must be established *a priori* to ensure patient safety. In this multi-institutional trial, a threshold criteria of observed abdominal or wound infection rate exceeding 15% would have led to study termination.

CONTINUOUS QUALITY IMPROVEMENT/CRITICAL CARE PATHWAYS

The foundation of CQI is monitoring and systematic evaluation to analyze information, identify potential deficiencies in care, and determine causes and avenues of improvement.[12] Standardized care can have a powerful impact on reducing cost, improving patient outcome, and facilitating research and the evaluation of new technologies and drugs. Any CQI monitoring and evaluation plan should include the following components: (1) the proper assignment of responsibility, (2) delineation of the scope of care based on the function and activities within the unit, (3) identification of important aspects of care that should be the focus of the review, (4) identification of appropriate and available indicators, (5) appropriate thresholds for evaluation, (6) methodologies for the collection and aggregation of data and its analysis, (7) evaluation of the care provided to determine whether an opportunity to improve care exists, (8) the initiation of actions (either improvement of care or the initiation of a different strategy) based on the monitoring and evaluation process, (9) assessment of actions conducted for improvement to determine if they were successful and care was improved, and (10) communication and integration of information to standardize the changes in the process and to maintain the improvements. In our surgical ICU, we conducted a CQI project to evaluate the efficacy and safety of our continuous positive airway pressure (CPAP) preextubation criterion (see Exhibit 13–2). Because the results did not exceed our threshold criterion (10% reintubation rate), we have continued to use this technique to evaluate extubation readiness. If CQI is properly conducted, it should meet the requirements of regulators and third-party payers for objective assessment of high-quality, cost-effective care.

Critical care pathways reflect coordination and documentation of care and show critical or key events (ie, consultations, diagnostic tests, activities, treatment, medications, diet, discharge planning, and teaching).[13] To develop a critical pathway, the steps are: (1) identify high-volume cases, (2) educate the staff, (3) convene a group of experts, (4) verify key incidents and time frames, (5) validate the data, (6) develop critical pathways, (7) reeducate the staff, and (8) implement the established pathways.

Unlike protocol manuals, guidelines set forth by regulatory agencies, or literature references that are written for a particular group of patients, critical pathways tie individual care plans of specialized groups into a team plan that provides a system of checks and balances that can reduce workload, promote quality care, and ultimately save time and money. It is important to include all disciplines that provide patient care in the development of critical pathways and use realistic time frames for thorough staff education regarding variance documentation. These activities should

---

Exhibit 13–2 Continuous Quality Improvement Project To Evaluate Preextubation Criteria

---

I. Important Aspects

The adequacy and timing of the weaning process is a measure of overall ICU assessment and care as well as the restoration of a satisfactory physiologic state for the patient. The timing of extubation can be used as an indicator balancing the risks that would be suffered by the patient if extubation was undertaken too early and overutilization of scarce resources if ventilatory support is excessively prolonged.

II. Assign Responsibility

- Physician Director: project design
- Fellows: clinical assessment, notes in chart, follow-up
- Attendings: daily evaluation of notes, discuss failures
- Staff: forms

continues

Exhibit 13–2 continued

III. Delineate Scope of Care

A. Types of patients
- Trauma: Operative and nonoperative
- Elective general surgery and specialties
- Emergency nontrauma, operated and nonoperated

B. Diagnosis and conditions: acute respiratory failure and airway management

C. Treatments/therapies
- Ventilatory support (ventilators, continuous positive airway pressure)
- Pulmonary toilet

D. Clinical activities: problem-oriented system evaluation

IV. Indicator

Reintubation within 48 hours of extubated patients who have the same disease and meet the following criteria:

1. Progress notes (SICU fellow) outlining general assessment of patient's condition and rationale for consideration of extubation
2. Trial when patient is breathing room air, continuous positive airway pressure + 5 cm H_2O: the spontaneous respiratory rate < 30/minute $PaO_2 > 55$ mm Hg, $PaCO_2 < 45$ mm Hg (previous eucapneic patient) and/or pHa > 7.35 (without metabolic acidosis).

V. Threshold

1. Prophylactic ventilation or early intervention: 5% failure rate
2. Advanced/late ARDS (adult respiratory distress syndrome) or preexisting chronic obstructive pulmonary disease (COPD): 20% failure rate.

VI. Methodology

1. Concurrent review of assessment note and data from CPAP room air trial by SICU attending physician during rounds.
2. Entry of demographic data, assessment and numerical data from CPAP room air trial in log by SICU fellow.
3. Daily chart review of patients extubated for the first two days with entry of reintubations in log book.
4. A 100-patient sample will be accumulated.

continues

Exhibit 13–2 continued

VII. Education

1. Review of all reintubations on morning teaching rounds. Comparison of criteria with established standards and determination, if possible, of reason for failure. If identified, it will be entered into the log.
2. Compilation of success and failure rate.
3. Compilation of factors leading to reintubation.

VIII. Action

The list of reasons for failure will be examined to identify failures in assessment, timing, or interpretation of data. Changing the weaning protocol would depend upon identification of such findings.

IX. Assessment of Actions for Improvement

A second 100-patient sample, incorporating changes and addressing problems identified in first sample, will be collected and compared to first sample.

X. Communication and Integration

1. If a change in population has occurred but the threshold is not exceeded, the characteristics that tend to increase the failure rate will be discussed with SICU attending physicians and fellows so that special attention is given to patients who are at higher risk for failure of extubation. A patient-care conference (composed of attending physicians, administrative nurses, fellows, respiratory therapists, and bedside nurses) will be held to discuss change in the unit population with all those involved in respiratory care.
2. If the threshold is exceeded and the criteria are changed, changing the weaning protocol will be necessary and these changes must be promulgated in the weaning protocol for SICU nurses and respiratory therapists. These changes will first be discussed at the staff administrative conference (SICU attending physicians, fellows, administrative nurses, and respiratory therapy supervisors); then after formulating a new protocol, this will be distributed to the fellows and communicated to the rest of the SICU staff in the patient-care conference.

be multidisciplinary and be part of the hospitalwide quality assessment/ improvement program.

STAFF EDUCATION

The primary purpose of developing and conducting research protocols is to improve patient outcomes. In the process, variability of practice is reduced and poor-quality care (with its increased complications, high costs, and poor outcomes) is often dramatically decreased. Education of the staff and important ancillary personnel is important to the success of the project. The expected benefits of outcomes research include: (1) achieving cost savings through expedited patient care, (2) minimizing duplication of services, (3) determining cost-benefit ratios through evaluation of services and patient care products, and (4) promoting collaborative practices and coordinating care to ensure the appropriate use of scarce resources, with the hope of decreasing length of stay and hospital readmission. Improving efficiency and diminishing unnecessary activity will decrease complications and have salutary effects. Physicians and nurses can return to thinking, assessing, and decision making instead of frenetically ordering, reacting, and intervening.

CASE DEMONSTRATION

Title

"Impact of in-line heat and moisture exchanger/airway filters versus heated humidification/tubing units on endotracheal tube occlusion and the incidence of ventilator-associated pneumonia"

Background

Humidification of anhydrous gases inspired from a mechanical ventilator through an endotracheal or tracheostomy tube has been proposed since the early 1950s, when these devices became readily accessible in the recovery room and intensive care areas. The two major approaches have been provision of exogenous humidification by various mechanical devices that are usually heated, or trapping and recycling endogenous heat and humidity from the exhaled gases with a heat and moisture exchanger (HME). One report using the heated humidifiers documented a ≥ 50% effective endotracheal lumen occlusion in about one of every five mechanically ventilated patients.[14] The cost of a heated humidification ventilator circuit, which is changed weekly, is comparable to that of a circuit using heat and moisture exchange units, when the HME is changed daily.

Objective

Evaluate the incidence and degree of endotracheal tube occlusion using the Pall BB100-F filter/heat and moisture exchanging unit (East Hills, New York) and the current method of using a heated humidification circuit. Demographics would suggest considerable cost savings in using the HME/filter if there is no difference between methods. The cost of the one heated humidification system is equivalent to the cost of using the HME for 7 days with daily changes of equipment. The mean duration of mechanical ventilation in our ICU is approximately 5 days.

Hypotheses

HMEs will have the same or decreased incidence of endotracheal tube occlusion. The incidence of ventilator-associated pneumonia (VAP) will be less because of reduced bidirectional contamination and/or endotoxin/bacterial removal. The costs of HME will be less than heated humidifiers.

Methods and Procedures

Mechanically ventilated patients were randomly assigned to receive one of the two humidification devices. The Pall BB100-F filter/HME unit was placed between the ventilator tubing "Y" and the Ballard closed suction system; the heated humidification circuit was used as current procedure dictates. HME exclusion criteria included pulmonary edema, excessive secretions, and hemoptysis. Mechanical ventilator tubing circuits were changed every 7 days, as per current practice. All patients were managed with partial ventilatory support as soon as feasible following admission to the ICU (pressure support ventilation to augment spontaneous respiratory activity and positive end-expiratory pressure/CPAP to maintain expiratory lung volume). Current clinical management practices for the ventilator were continued. Upon extubation or endotracheal tube removal, the tube was cut at the point of apparent maximal occlusion and quantified into quartiles: 0–25%, 25–50%, 50–75%, or 75–100% at point of maximal occlusion as determined by the extubator. Patients underwent bronchoscopic examination if there was suspicion of endotracheal tube obstruction. If there was obstruction, the endotracheal tube was changed or the patient extubated. If bronchoscopic examination of the endotracheal tube was negative, these patients were followed until the preextubation trial was completed and the patient extubated.

Data Collection

The following information was obtained at the time of extubation or change of endotracheal tube. Percentage of occlusion, if any, was recorded. Duration of mechanical ventilation was used to calculate the cost of disposable tubing and humidification system components. Incidence of nosocomial pneumonia and the percentage of occlusion, if any, were recorded. Duration of mechanical ventilation was used to calculate the cost of disposable tubing and humidification system components.

Statistical Analysis

This was an unpaired case study for artificial airway partial occlusion and pneumonia incidence. Retrospective analysis revealed a 30% incidence of VAP. Viewing a 15% change as significant, and choosing a 5% alpha error and 5% beta error, it was necessary to enroll 100 patients per group.

Study Clarification

No attempt was made to alter in any fashion the current clinical practice or to modify the prevalence of certain procedures such as "breaking" the circuit to bag and suction the patient manually. The assumption was that the incidence of these occurrences remains the same.

Findings and Conclusions

Report of Results

Findings of this study were reported to the appropriate departmental participants for dispersal and submitted for scientific review and publication. The results were also used to suggest and evaluate future investigations into modifications of existing clinical practices.

Results

Three patients were dropped from the study to be placed on an ultra-high-frequency ventilator; an additional three were dropped for clinical reasons (hemoptysis secondary to multiple stab wounds, pulmonary edema, and presentation to the ICU with copious secretions). Of the patients who remained in the study, there were no documented occlusions of the HME device, no impacted secretions, and no cases of hypothermia.

Of the 100 patients in the heated-wire humidifier group, there were 20 cases of community-acquired pneumonia (ie, new or progressive infiltrate on chest X-ray, productive sputum, positive tracheobronchial culture within 3 days of ventilation). There were 16 cases of nosocomial VAP after 3 days.

The HME group exhibited the same incidence number of community-acquired pneumonia (19 patients out of 100), but this group had only 7 cases of nosocomial VAP. Distribution of pathogens cultured showed no differences between the heated-wire humidifier and HME groups. We observed a reduction in circuit costs from $2,880 to $1,775 per patient for the same 100 patients in each group. There were no differences between the groups in average duration of ventilation or total number of ventilator days. The community-acquired pneumonia rates per 100 ventilator days were comparable between groups; the nosocomial VAP rate per 1000 ventilator days was significantly reduced with the HME.

Comparison between the heated-wire wick humidifier and the HME showed no difference in duration of ventilation for those patients without pneumonia; they were ventilated about 2.5 days. Patients with community-acquired pneumonia were ventilated about 8 days (median = 7.5 to 8.0 days). Patients with nosocomial VAP were ventilated an average of 16 days, with a median of 15 to 16 days. One patient in the HME group was ventilated for 55 days, accounting for the apparent difference in mean values and larger standard deviation. There were no observed differences in endotracheal tube obstruction or resistive work of breathing. In summary, a 44% reduction in nosocomial VAP was achieved with the use of HME filters.

SUMMARY

The physician must become an aggressive proponent of cost-efficiency in order to enhance the quality and efficiency of patient care at all levels of the delivery continuum. Physicians must demand that future advances in pharmacologic and device technology parallel clinical needs and show a measurable benefit to patient outcomes, reduce length of stay, or reduce patient costs. Physician leaders must define and diligently measure their own progress, implementing and evaluating outcomes of research and standardized care protocols. Physicians must learn the importance of protocols and research to improve the efficiency of the utilization of resources. For virtually every management decision, the physician must explicitly identify, weigh, and balance all available treatment alternatives; weigh the benefits against the risks and costs; and factor in ethical, societal, and legal considerations. Accordingly, high-quality systematic reviews and outcomes-driven research are being used to guide clinical care, strengthening the link between research and improved outcomes. In this way, we can respond to Fuchs's exhortation that "physicians consider the possibility of contributing more by doing less."[15(p 3)] We must first contribute more by achieving a greater understanding of the medical care process.

REFERENCES

1. Cook DJ, Sibbald WJ, Vincent JL, et al. Evidence based critical care medicine: What is it and what can it do for us? *Crit Care Med.* 1996;24:334–337.

2. Shapiro BA, Warren J, Egol AB, et al. Practice parameters for sustained neuromuscular blockade in the adult critically ill patient: An executive summary. *Crit Care Med.* 1995;23:1601–1605.

3. Kirton OC, Civetta JM. Setting objectives: Perspective for care. In: Civetta JM, Taylor RW, Kirby RR, eds. *Critical Care*, 3rd ed. Philadelphia: JB Lippincott Raven; 1997;2:21–34.

4. Wedderburn, R, Kirton OC, Shatz DV, et al. Management of supraventricular tach-yarrhythmias in the critically-ill surgical patient. *Crit Care Med.* 1993;22:A99.

5. Civetta JM, Hudson-Civetta JA, Dion L. Duration of illness affects catheter-related infection and bacteremia. *Program and Abstracts of the 27th Interscience Conference on Antimicrobial Agents and Chemotherapy.* 1987;69:1141.

6. Maki DG, Weise CE, Sarafin HW. A semi-quantitative culture method for identifying intravenous-catheter-related infection. *N Engl J Med.* 1977;296:1305–1309.

7. Ball ES, Hudson-Civetta J, Civetta JM. Re-evaluation of insertion and guidewire exchange (GWX) protocols' effectiveness and validity. *Crit Care Med.* 1995;23:A250.

8. Clemence MA, Jernigan JA, Titus MA, et al. A study of an antiseptic impregnated central venous catheter for prevention of bloodstream infection. *Program and Abstract Proceedings of the 33rd Interscience Conference on Antimicrobial Agents and Chemotherapy.* 1993;72:1023.

9. Kirton OC, Banner MJ, Axelrad A, et al. Detection of unsuspected imposed work of breathing: Case reports. *Crit Care Med.* 1993;21:790–795.

10. Kirton OC, DeHaven CB, Morgan JP, et al. Elevated imposed work of breathing masquerading as ventilator weaning intolerance. *Chest.* 1995;108:1021–1025.

11. DeHaven CB, Kirton OC, Morgan JP, et al. Breathing measurement reduces false negative classification of tachypneic extubation trial failures. *Crit Care Med.* 1996;24:976–980.

12. Rifkin M. Quality assessment and improvement in the ICU: Its influence on bedside practice. In: Civetta JM, Taylor RW, Kirby RR. *Critical Care.* Philadelphia: JB Lippincott Co; 1992:1899–1916.

13. Nelson MS. Critical pathways in the emergency department. *J Emerg Nurs.* 1993;19:110–114.

14. DeHaven B, Kirton OC, Morgan J, et al. The use of a bacterial filter/heat moisture exchanger does not impact imposed work of breathing during mechanical ventilation. *Crit Care Med.* 1994;32:A119.

15. Fuchs VR. A more effective, efficient, and equitable system. *West J Med.* 1976;125:3.

Index